INTERCOLLEGIATE MRCS: 300 SINGLE BEST ANSWER QUESTIONS IN APPLIED BASIC SCIENCES

Shahzad G. Raja

BSc., MBBS, MRCS

Specialist Registrar Cardiothoracic Surgery

Department of Cardiothoracic Surgery

Glasgow Royal Infirmary

Glasgow

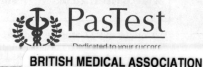

PasTest

Dedicated to your success

First Published 2006

ISBN: 1 905635 060
ISBN: 978 1 905635 061

A catalogue record for this book is available from the British Library.

The information contained within this book was obtained by the author from reliable sources. However, while every effort has been made to ensure its accuracy, no responsibility for loss, damage or injury occasioned to any person acting or refraining from action as a result of information contained herein can be accepted by the publishers or author.

Every effort has been made to contact holders of copyright to obtain permission to reproduce copyright material. However, if any have been inadvertently overlooked, the publisher will be pleased to make the necessary arrangements at the first opportunity.

PasTest Revision Books and Intensive Courses

PasTest has been established in the field of postgraduate medical education since 1972, providing revision books and intensive study courses for doctors preparing for their professional examinations.

Books and courses are available for the following specialties:

MRCGP, MRCP Parts 1 and 2, MRCPCH Parts 1 and 2, MRCPsych, MRCS, MRCOG Parts 1 and 2, DRCOG, DCH, FRCA, PLAB Parts 1 and 2, Dental Students, Dentists and Dental Nurses.

For further details contact:

PasTest, Freepost, Knutsford, Cheshire WA16 7BR

Tel: 01565 752000   **Fax: 01565 650264**

www.pastest.co.uk   **enquires@pastest.co.uk**

Text prepared by Carnegie Book Production, Lancaster

Printed and bound by MPG Books Ltd, Bodmin, Cornwall

CONTENTS

ACKNOWLEDGEMENTS

To my parents who made me what I am today and taught me the difference between good intentions and good deeds.

To my loving wife, Irfana, for her unwavering support and love in all my endeavours.

To my son, Roheen, who provides me with limitless pleasure and gives me my purpose in life.

INTRODUCTION

Commencing in September 2006 traditional true/false multiple choice questions in the Part I paper (Applied Basic Sciences) of the Intercollegiate MRCS will be gradually replaced by questions that will have a 'Single Best Answer' or 'Best of Five' style format. This change has been prompted by the major changes in postgraduate medical education currently occurring in the United Kingdom. **Intercollegiate MRCS: 300 Single Best Answer Questions in Applied Basic Sciences** has been written with the primary objective of providing MRCS candidates with a series of questions that will prepare them for this new format. As the new format of the Part I paper de-emphasises the traditional basic science disciplines and stresses the integrated approach, this book contains a substantial number of patient-based questions or clinical vignettes that will enable prospective candidates to test their ability to integrate key basic science concepts with relevant clinical problems.

In keeping with the ethos of the examination, the book focuses intensively on the application of the basic sciences (anatomy, physiology, pathology, microbiology and pharmacology) to the management of surgical patients. Much emphasis has been placed on the physiological and pharmacological basis of post-operative care, ITU care, as well as the anatomical basis of commonly undertaken ward procedures and surgical operations.

The book is split into three main sections, namely Anatomy, Physiology and Pathology, with each section containing 100 questions. Each question has been carefully formulated to cover a given section of the Intercollegiate MRCS syllabus in Applied Basic Sciences. Most major sections of the syllabus are dealt with and answers with detailed explanations are provided to enable the candidates to develop their understanding of each topic. Several different subtypes of 'Single Best Answer Questions' have been included in this book so as to offer effective exam practice and guide candidates through their revision and exam technique. These include *clinical case questions/clinical vignettes* (basic science in clinical clothing), *positively worded questions* that ask candidates to select the answer that is 'most likely' to be true, *two-step/double jump questions* that require several cognitive steps to arrive at a correct answer and last but not least *factual recall true/false questions* that probe for basic recall of facts.

I hope that you have as much pleasure in attempting these questions as I had in preparing them.

Shahzad G. Raja

BSc MBBS MRCS

THE INTERCOLLEGIATE MEMBERSHIP OF THE ROYAL COLLEGE OF SURGEONS (MRCS) EXAMINATION

This new examination was agreed by, and is common to, the Surgical Royal Colleges of Great Britain and Ireland. It replaces the MRCS Eng, MRCS Glas, AFRCS Ed, and MRCS I, which previously had different formats, papers, pass rates, and syllabi. The intercollegiate exam was introduced in October 2004 and the old examinations were phased out simultaneously. It forms part of the requirement for the Certificate of Completion of Basic Surgical Training (CCBST) which includes:

- Possession of an acceptable primary medical qualification (MBChB)
- Pass in all parts of the MRCS intercollegiate examination
- Successful completion of 24 months' training in recognised posts from defined specialities
- Completion of mandatory courses

The CCBST is the minimum requirement for applicants for a Higher Surgical Training rotation in surgery. Successful applicants are awarded a National Training Number and become specialist registrars in their chosen surgical speciality. Higher Surgical Training culminates in the Certificate of Completion of Specialist Training (CCST) which, in General Surgery at least, is awarded only after passing the 'exit' or Intercollegiate Examination (ICE). This CCST enables the holder to take up a post as an independent practitioner (consultant) in their speciality.

Eligibility for the intercollegiate MRCS

- Candidates must possess an acceptable primary medical qualification (MBChB)
- Candidates may apply to sit Part 1 at any time after gaining their primary medical qualification (eg during house jobs)
- Candidates must have commenced Basic Surgical Training (BST) before entering Part 2 of the exam
- Candidates may sit Part 1 and Part 2 in any order, and with any of the British and Irish colleges. Candidates may sit Part 1 and Part 2 at different colleges
- Candidates may re-sit Part 1 and Part 2 as many times as they wish

Candidates have a time limit of three-and-a-half years in which to complete all parts of the examination dating from their first attempt at Part 2, even if they sit Part 2 before Part 1. Three-and-a-half years after sitting Part 2, if candidates have not passed both the clinical and the viva sections of Part 3, they will never be allowed to re-sit any part of the examination.

STRUCTURE OF THE INTERCOLLEGIATE MRCS

PART 1 Applied Basic Sciences Multiple True False paper to be gradually replaced with Single Best Answer Questions commencing September 2006 (Duration: 3 hours)

PART 2 Clinical Problem Solving Extended Matching Questions paper (Duration: 3 hours)

- Held three times a year simultaneously worldwide
- Candidates must pass both papers before proceeding to Part 3

PART 3 (two components)

1. Oral component

This consists of three 20-minute vivas on:

- Applied surgical anatomy and operative surgery
- Applied physiology and critical care
- Applied surgical pathology and principles of surgery

Candidates must pass the overall oral component before proceeding to the clinical component.

2. Clinical component

There are six bays in total: four clinical bays and two communication bays.

The four 15-minute clinical bays require candidates to examine, diagnose, elicit physical signs and show that they are familiar with the treatment of patients. These four bays are:

- Trauma and orthopaedics
- Vascular
- Breast, skin, head and neck
- Trunk, groin and scrotum

The two bays of communication test skills over a total of 30 minutes

- Taking a history to reach a diagnosis
- Giving information to patients, relatives, or other healthcare professionals

Candidates who fail the clinical component will not be required to re-take the oral component, but will have to pass the clinical component within three-and-a-half years of sitting Part 2.

The structure, timing, regulations and requirements for these examinations are constantly changing as the exams are updated. The above outline was accurate at the time of writing, but you should not rely on this or any other printed or verbal information because it may be out of date as soon as it is reaches you. Contact your Royal College; their website is often the most up-to-date source of information.

USEFUL ADDRESSES

The Royal College of Surgeons of England

35–43 Lincoln's Inn Fields
London WC2A 3PE

Tel: 0207 869 6281 (+ 44 20 7 405 3474)

http:/www.rcseng.ac.uk/

The Royal College of Surgeons of Edinburgh

Information Section
Adamson Centre
3 Hill Place
Edinburgh EH8 9DS

Tel: 0131 668 9222 (+ 44 131 668 9222)

http:/www.rcsed.ac.uk/

The Royal College of Physicians and Surgeons of Glasgow

232–242 Vincent Street
Glasgow G2 5RJ

Tel: 0141 221 6072 (+ 44 141 221 6072)

http:/www.rcpsglasg.ac.uk/

The Royal College of Surgeons in Ireland

123 St Stephens Green
Dublin 2, Ireland

Tel: +353 1 402 2223 (+ 353 1 402 2100)

http:/www.rcsi.ie/

ABBREVIATIONS

A&E	accident and emergency department
ACE	angiotensin-converting enzyme
ADH	antidiuretic hormone
AFP	α-fetoprotein
AIDS	acquired immune deficiency syndrome
AJCC	American Joint Committee on Cancer
ARDS	acute respiratory distress syndrome
ARF	acute renal failure
ATN	acute tubular necrosis
AV	atrioventricular
cAMP	cyclic adenosine monophosphate
CCK	cholecystokinin
CEA	carcinoembryonic antigen
CN	cranial nerve
CNS	central nervous system
CO	cardiac output
COPD	chronic obstructive pulmonary disease
COX-2	cyclo-oxygenase-2
CPK	creatine kinase
CRP	C-reactive protein
CSF	cerebrospinal fluid
CT	computed tomography
CVP	central venous pressure
DHT	5β-dihydrotestosterone
D_{LCO}	carbon monoxide diffusing capacity
2,3-DPG	2,3-diphosphoglycerate
DPL	diagnostic peritoneal lavage/tap
DVT	deep venous thrombosis
ECF	extracellular fluid
EDV	end-diastolic volume
EF	ejection fraction
ESD	end-systolic volume
ESR	erythrocyte sedimentation rate

FEV$_1$	forced expiratory volume in 1 s
FGF	fibroblast growth factor
FNA	fine-needle aspiration
FRC	functional residual capacity
FVC	forced vital capacity
GFR	glomerular filtration rate
GH	growth hormone
GM-CSF	granulocyte–macrophage colony-stimulating factor
GORD	gastro-oesophageal reflux disease
GVHD	graft-versus-host disease
HBV	hepatitis B virus
β-hCG	β-human chorionic gonadotrophin
HDL	high-density lipoprotein
HIV	human immunodeficiency virus
HLA	human leukocyte antigen
HR	heart rate
ICU	intensive care unit
IP$_3$	inositol triphosphate
IVC	inferior vena cava
JGA	juxtaglomerular apparatus
JVP	jugular venous pulse (pressure)
LAP	left atrial pressure
LDH	lactate dehydrogenase
LDL	low-density lipoprotein
LMW	low-molecular-weight
MAC	membrane attack complex
MAP	mean arterial pressure
MCH	mean corpuscular haemoglobin
MCHC	mean corpuscular haemoglobin concentration
MCV	mean corpuscular volume
MEN	multiple endocrine neoplasia
MIP	macrophage inflammatory protein
MPAP	mean pulmonary artery pressure
MRI	magnetic resonance imaging
MRSA	methicillin-resistant *Staphylococcus aureus*
MSSA	methicillin-sensitive *Staphylococcus aureus*

NK	natural killer
NSAID	non-steroidal anti-inflammatory drug
NSGCT	non-seminomatous germ-cell tumour
PAF	platelet-activating factor
PAH	p-aminohippuric acid
PAWP	pulmonary artery wedge pressure
$P\text{CO}_2$	partial pressure of carbon dioxide
PE	pulmonary embolism
PNS	parasympathetic nervous system
$P\text{O}_2$	partial pressure of oxygen
RBCs	red blood cells
RF	rheumatic fever
RPF	renal plasma flow
RV	residual volume
SA	sinoatrial
SAA	serum amyloid A
SIADH	syndrome of inappropriate ADH secretion
SLE	systemic lupus erythematosus
SV	stroke volume
$S\text{vo}_2$	mixed venous oxygen saturation
SVR	systemic vascular resistance
T_3	triiodothyronine
T_4	thyroxine
TB	tuberculosis
TGF	transforming growth factor
Th1	T-helper cell
TLC	total lung capacity
TNM	tumour, node, metastases
tPA	tissue plasminogen activator
TPN	total parenteral nutrition
TRH	thyroid-releasing hormone
TSH	thyroid-stimulating hormone
UICC	Union Internationale Contre le Cancer
UTI	urinary tract infection
VC	vital capacity
VIP	vasoactive poplypeptide

QUESTIONS

SECTION 1:
ANATOMY – QUESTIONS

For each question given below choose the SINGLE BEST option.

1.1   **A 22-year-old man is stabbed in the axilla. There is profuse bleeding from the axillary artery. Which of the following statements about the axillary artery is true?**

   A   It originates from the arch of the aorta

   B   It gives origin to the thoracoacromial artery

   C   It has the lateral thoracic artery as its first branch

   D   It divides into radial and ulnar arteries in the cubital fossa

   E   It provides no blood supply to the humerus

1.2   **A man stabbed in a bar fight suffers a penetrating wound through the anterior axillary fold, with resulting damage to one of the main terminal branches of the brachial plexus. Clinical examination in the accident and emergency department (A&E) revealed a significant weakening of flexion of the elbow. The other effect to be expected is:**

   A   Loss of cutaneous sensation on the tips of several fingers

   B   Loss of cutaneous sensation just on the anterolateral surface of the forearm

   C   Just weakening of flexion at the shoulder

   D   Weakening of flexion at the shoulder and loss of cutaneous sensation on the anterolateral surface of the arm

   E   Weakening of flexion at the shoulder and loss of cutaneous sensation on the anterolateral surface of the forearm

anatomy

1.3 **After a road traffic accident a young man is noticed to have suffered injury to the lower subscapular nerve. Injury to the lower subscapular nerve will affect the function of:**

○ A Teres major muscle

○ B Teres minor muscle

○ C Deltoid muscle

○ D Supraspinatus muscle

○ E Infraspinatus muscle

1.4 **A 62-year-old woman has a loop of bowel herniating into the femoral canal. Which of the following statements best describes the femoral canal?**

○ A It is superficial to the inguinal ligament

○ B It transmits the obturator nerve

○ C It is the medial compartment of the femoral sheath

○ D It transmits the femoral artery

○ E It is lateral to the femoral nerve

1.5 **Clinical examination of a patient with a diabetic ulcer in the anterior midline of the ankle region elicited loss of cutaneous sensation on the dorsal surface of the foot. Which nerve was most probably damaged?**

○ A Femoral

○ B Lateral sural cutaneous

○ C Saphenous

○ D Sural

○ E Superficial peroneal

1.6 **A 20-year-old man presents in A&E with features suggestive of common peroneal nerve injury. The common peroneal nerve is most commonly injured:**

○ A Where it emerges below the piriformis muscle

○ B At the site where it divides into the superficial and deep peroneal nerves

○ C Where it leaves the sciatic nerve in the popliteal fossa

○ D As it branches into the head of the biceps femoris

○ E Just behind the head of the fibula

1.7 **A 2-year-old baby developed chylothorax as a result of iatrogenic injury to the thoracic duct at the time of surgery to correct a congenital cardiac defect. Which of the following statements about the thoracic duct is true?**

○ A It returns lymph from the convex surface of the liver

○ B It extends from the fifth lumbar vertebra to the root of the neck

○ C It enters the thorax through the aortic hiatus of the diaphragm

○ D It ends by opening into the angle of junction of the right subclavian vein with the right internal jugular vein

○ E It has no valves to ensure smooth flow of lymph

1.8 **A patient with acute anal fissure has severe pain. The pain sensations in this condition are transmitted by:**

○ A The superior rectal nerve

○ B The inferior rectal nerve

○ C The pelvic splanchnic nerve

○ D The perineal nerve

○ E The posterior scrotal nerve

anatomy

3

1.9 A junior house officer is assisting repair of an inguinal hernia for the first time. The consultant asks him to identify the roof of the inguinal canal. The roof of the inguinal canal is formed by:

○ A   Aponeurosis of the external oblique

○ B   A lacunar ligament

○ C   Reflected inguinal ligament

○ D   Union of the transversalis fascia with the inguinal ligament

○ E   Arched fibres of internal oblique and transversus abdominis

1.10 During mobilisation of the descending aorta for repair of coarctation of aorta, a surgeon accidentally cuts the first aortic intercostal artery. Which of the following structures might be deprived of its main source of blood supply?

○ A   First posterior intercostal space

○ B   First anterior intercostal space

○ C   Right bronchus

○ D   Left bronchus

○ E   Fibrous pericardium

1.11 The thoracoabdominal diaphragm is pierced by three large apertures for the passage of the aorta, vena cava and oesophagus between the thorax and abdomen. Which of the following statements about these openings in the diaphragm is true?

○ A   The aortic hiatus is the highest and most anterior of the large apertures

○ B   The aortic hiatus is in the central tendon

○ C   The oesophageal hiatus is at the level of the ninth thoracic vertebra

○ D   The vena caval foramen is quadrilateral in shape

○ E   The vena caval foramen transmits some branches of the left phrenic nerve

1.12 **A patient with an ulcerative carcinoma of the posterior third of the tongue presented in A&E with arterial bleeding from the lesion. Which of the following arteries was involved?**

- A   Deep lingual
- B   Dorsal lingual
- C   Facial
- D   Sublingual
- E   Tonsillar

1.13 **After a myocardial infarction a patient underwent coronary angiography, which showed a blockade in the left coronary artery. Which of the following statements about the left coronary artery is true?**

- A   It is smaller than the right coronary artery
- B   It gives off a large marginal branch
- C   It continues to the apex of the heart as the posterior descending branch
- D   It supplies both ventricles
- E   It supplies the whole of the conducting system of the heart

1.14 **A 40-year-old man with dysphagia underwent oesophagoscopy, which revealed an exophytic growth in the abdominal part of the oesophagus. Which of the following statements about the abdominal portion of the oesophagus is true?**

- A   It lies in the oesophageal groove on the posterior surface of the right lobe of the liver
- B   It is about 3.5 cm in length
- C   It is supplied by the left gastric branch of the coeliac artery
- D   It is completely intraperitoneal
- E   It is mainly innervated by the left phrenic nerve

1.15 **You are performing your first appendicectomy. Initially, on entering the right iliac fossa you do not find the appendix. However, you do not panic because you know that you can quickly locate it by:**

- ○ A Palpating the ileocaecal valve and looking just above it
- ○ B Looking at the confluence of the taeniae coli
- ○ C Following the course of the right colic artery
- ○ D Removing the right layer of the mesentery of the jejunoileum
- ○ E Palpating and inspecting the pelvic brim

1.16 **A 26-year-old woman developed Bell's palsy of the facial nerve after a herpes simplex viral infection. Which of the following statements about the facial nerve is true?**

- ○ A It supplies the muscles of mastication
- ○ B It contains some sympathetic motor fibres, which constitute the vasodilator nerves of the parotid gland
- ○ C It is a pure motor nerve
- ○ D It has a sensory part that contains the fibres of taste for the anterior two-thirds of the tongue
- ○ E It arises from the midbrain

1.17 **You are assisting exploratory laparotomy for a firearm injury involving the second part of the duodenum. On entering the peritoneal cavity, which of the following structures will you see anterior to the second part of the duodenum?**

- ○ A Right colic flexure
- ○ B Hilum of right kidney
- ○ C Renal vessels
- ○ D Inferior vena cava
- ○ E Psoas muscle

1.18 **The cystic artery supplying the gallbladder is usually a branch of**:

○   A   The gastroduodenal artery

○   B   The right gastric artery

○   C   The hepatic proper artery

○   D   The right hepatic artery

○   E   The left hepatic artery

1.19 **The femoral triangle is bounded laterally by the medial border of**:

○   A   Sartorius

○   B   Iliacus

○   C   Psoas major

○   D   Pectineus

○   E   Adductor brevis

1.20 **After a street fight a young man arrived in A&E with a stab wound on the right thigh involving the adductor canal. Which of the following structures is most likely to be injured in this patient?**

○   A   The popliteal artery

○   B   The saphenous vein

○   C   The sural nerve

○   D   The obturator artery

○   E   The nerve to vastus medialis

anatomy

1.21 During surgery on the right submandibular gland the lingual nerve gets injured. Postoperatively, the patient will complain of:

○ A Deviation of the tongue to the right

○ B Deviation of the tongue to the left

○ C Loss of taste sensation over the anterior two-thirds of the right side of the tongue

○ D Loss of taste sensation over the posterior one-third of the right side of the tongue

○ E Loss of general sensation over the posterior one-third of the right side of the tongue

1.22 The superior gluteal artery typically exits the pelvis:

○ A Above the lumbosacral trunk

○ B Between the lumbosacral trunk and S1 nerve

○ C Between the S1 and S2 nerves

○ D Between the S2 and S3 nerves

○ E Through the lesser sciatic foramen

1.23 An injury involving the anatomical snuffbox is likely to damage:

○ A The radial nerve

○ B The median nerve

○ C The radial artery

○ D The ulnar nerve

○ E The ulnar artery

1.24 **A patient presents in A&E with a bullet wound that has severed the musculocutaneous nerve at its origin. On clinical examination which of the following will be elicited?**

○ A   Action of supinator

○ B   Action of brachialis

○ C   Action of coracobrachialis

○ D   Action of biceps brachii

○ E   Sensations over lower two-thirds of the dorsolateral surface of the forearm

1.25 **During cranial nerve examination, the integrity of the right trochlear nerve can be tested by asking the patient to look:**

○ A   Towards the nose in a horizontal plane

○ B   Inwards, towards the nose and downwards

○ C   Laterally in a horizontal plane

○ D   Outwards, away from the nose and downwards

○ E   Inwards, towards the nose and upwards

1.26 **Clinical examination of a patient complaining of frequent episodes of aspiration of fluid into her lungs after subtotal thyroidectomy revealed that the area of the piriform recess above the vocal fold of the larynx was numb. This is the result of intraoperative injury to:**

○ A   The lingual nerve

○ B   The recurrent laryngeal nerve

○ C   The external branch of the superior pharyngeal nerve

○ D   The hypoglossal nerve

○ E   The internal branch of the superior laryngeal nerve

anatomy

1.27 **A patient with enlarged deep cervical lymph nodes as a result of a metastatic carcinoma complains of hoarseness. The hoarse voice is caused by enlarged nodes pressing:**

○ A The external branch of the superior laryngeal nerve

○ B The internal branch of the superior laryngeal nerve

○ C The recurrent laryngeal branch of vagus

○ D The nerve to the cricothyroid muscle

○ E The pharyngeal branch of the glossopharyngeal nerve

1.28 **A patient presents in A&E with a laceration on the temporal region, resulting in loss of sensation from the temporal region and loss of secretory function of the parotid gland. The laceration has severed:**

○ A The chorda tympani

○ B The posterior deep temporal nerve

○ C The facial nerve

○ D The auriculotemporal nerve

○ E The great auricular nerve

1.29 **A 16-year-old boy with left-sided indirect inguinal hernia presents in A&E with features of large bowel obstruction resulting from the hernia. The intestinal segment most likely to be involved in this obstruction is:**

○ A The caecum

○ B The ascending colon

○ C The descending colon

○ D The rectum

○ E The sigmoid colon

1.30 **While walking barefooted in the garden a housewife was injured with a broken piece of glass that penetrated the plantar aponeurosis and injured muscles in the first layer. Which of the following muscles is most likely to be affected?**

○　A　Abductor digiti minimi

○　B　Flexor accessorius

○　C　Lumbricales

○　D　Adductor hallucis

○　E　Interossei

1.31 **The posterior mediastinal structure most closely applied to the posterior surface of the pericardial sac is:**

○　A　The aorta

○　B　The oesophagus

○　C　The azygos vein

○　D　The thoracic duct

○　E　The trachea

1.32 **The muscle of the forearm innervated by both median and ulnar nerves is:**

○　A　Flexor carpi ulnaris

○　B　Flexor digitorum superficialis

○　C　Flexor digitorum profundus

○　D　Pronator quadratus

○　E　Flexor pollicis longus

anatomy

1.33 The hand muscle likely to be affected by compression of the median nerve in the carpal tunnel is:

○ A   Flexor pollicis brevis

○ B   Opponens digiti minimi

○ C   Flexor pollicis longus

○ D   Dorsal interossei

○ E   Palmar interossei

1.34 The carpal bone most commonly dislocated by a fall on an outstretched hand is:

○ A   The trapezoid

○ B   The lunate

○ C   The scaphoid

○ D   The hamate

○ E   The capitate

1.35 A 45-year-old woman with carcinoma of the breast has enlarged axillary lymph nodes. About 75% of the lymph draining the breast goes to:

○ A   The deltopectoral lymph nodes

○ B   The lateral axillary lymph nodes

○ C   The parasternal lymph nodes

○ D   The subscapular lymph nodes

○ E   The central axillary lymph nodes

1.36 **After a right-sided mastectomy a woman complains of winging of the scapula. The most likely nerve to be injured in this operation is:**

- A The long thoracic nerve
- B The accessory nerve
- C The lateral pectoral nerve
- D The phrenic nerve
- E The vagus nerve

1.37 **A patient with aortic dissection suffered infarction of the lower spinal cord as a result of extension of the dissection into the artery of Adamkiewicz. Which of the following statements best describes this artery?**

- A It is also known as the artery of lumbar enlargement
- B It is a radicular artery in the lower thoracic or upper lumbar region
- C It is most frequently found on the right side
- D It has extensive anastomoses on the surface of the sacral spinal cord
- E It passes through foramina in the bodies of the vertebrae to reach the cord

1.38 **A superficial cut on the ulnar side of forearm is most likely to damage:**

- A The basilic vein
- B The cephalic vein
- C The median cubital vein
- D The median antebrachial vein
- E The ulnar vein

anatomy

1.39 **A patient with fracture of the surgical neck of humerus is most likely to injure:**

○   A   The subscapular artery

○   B   The circumflex scapular artery

○   C   The posterior humeral circumflex artery

○   D   The radial recurrent artery

○   E   The brachial artery

1.40 **A fracture of the sustentaculum tali will adversely affect the function of:**

○   A   Flexor digitorum longus

○   B   Flexor hallucis longus

○   C   Fibularis longus

○   D   Tibialis anterior

○   E   Tibialis posterior

1.41 **A 16-year-old girl stepped on a broken piece of glass while walking barefoot and severed the lateral plantar nerve in her left foot. The lateral plantar nerve is a branch of:**

○   A   The tibial nerve

○   B   The sural nerve

○   C   The deep peroneal nerve

○   D   The saphenous nerve

○   E   The femoral nerve

1.42 **Scissor gait is caused by overactive adduction of the thigh. The nerve responsible for this abnormality is:**

○ A   The femoral nerve

○ B   The tibial nerve

○ C   The saphenous nerve

○ D   The inferior gluteal nerve

○ E   The obturator nerve

1.43 **Avascular necrosis of the femoral head after fracture of the neck of the femur results from interruption of:**

○ A   The lateral circumflex femoral artery

○ B   The internal pudendal artery

○ C   The first perforating branch of the deep femoral artery

○ D   The medial circumflex femoral artery

○ E   The descending genicular artery

1.44 **A patient with a bleeding gastric ulcer of the lesser curvature of the stomach is scoped to identify the source of bleeding. The vessel most likely to be involved will be:**

○ A   The left gastric artery

○ B   The left gastroepiploic artery

○ C   The right gastroepiploic artery

○ D   The gastroduodenal artery

○ E   The short gastric arteries

anatomy

1.45 At the time of splenectomy, the tail of pancreas must be identified in:

○ A The transverse mesocolon

○ B The gastrocolic ligament

○ C The gastrosplenic ligament

○ D The phrenicolic ligament

○ E The splenorenal ligament

1.46 Of the organs listed below the one that is covered entirely by visceral peritoneum is:

○ A The pancreas

○ B The spleen

○ C The adrenal gland

○ D The kidney

○ E The duodenum

1.47 You have scrubbed up for the first time with your consultant who is performing exploratory laparotomy for a mass in the right upper quadrant of the abdomen. You are asked by your consultant to identify the third part of the duodenum. Which of the following features will enable you to correctly identify this?

○ A It is 10 cm long

○ B It begins at the left side of the upper border of the fourth lumbar vertebra

○ C It is crossed by the superior mesenteric vessels

○ D It is 2 cm medial to the mesentery of the small bowel

○ E Its upper surface is in relation with the tail of the pancreas

1.48 Compared with the ileum, the jejunum:

○　A　Is narrow

○　B　Is thinner

○　C　Is less vascular

○　D　Has larger villi

○　E　Has more numerous Peyer's patches

1.49 While performing exploratory laparotomy, which of the following features will help you to distinguish the ileum from the jejunum?

○　A　It possesses numerous circular folds

○　B　It chiefly occupies the umbilical and left iliac regions

○　C　It has larger and more numerous aggregated lymph nodes

○　D　It is more vascular

○　E　It is retroperitoneal

1.50 A 62-year-old with chronic alcohol problems developed obstructive jaundice as a result of a carcinoma in the head of the pancreas. Which of the following statements about the head of the pancreas is true?

○　A　It is lodged within the curve of the jejunum

○　B　It is posteriorly related to the superior mesenteric vessels

○　C　It is posteriorly related to the root of the mesentery

○　D　It is posteriorly related to the common bile duct

○　E　It is anteriorly related to the right crus of diaphragm

anatomy

1.51 Embryologically, as the pancreas develops in two parts it has two ducts. Which of the following statements about the main pancreatic duct is true?

○ A It is also called the duct of Wirsung

○ B It extends transversely from right to left through the substance of the pancreas

○ C It has the common bile duct on its left side as it leaves the head of pancreas

○ D It ends by an orifice common to it and the common bile duct in the third part of the duodenum

○ E It is a derivative of the dorsal pancreatic bud

1.52 The anterior surface of the right kidney is related to:

○ A The medial lumbocostal arch

○ B The iliohypogastric nerve

○ C The ilioinguinal nerve

○ D The last thoracic nerve

○ E The right colic flexure

1.53 During exploratory laparotomy, which of the following features will enable you to identify the superior surface of the liver?

○ A It is made up of the right lobe only

○ B It is covered by peritoneum only along the line of attachment of the falciform ligament

○ C It is related to the seventh and eighth costal cartilages on the left side

○ D It is related to the fifth to eighth ribs on the right side

○ E It is in contact with the pylorus in the angle between the diverging rib cartilage of opposite sides

1.54 **A 45-year-old man with Barrett's oesophagus underwent oesophagoscopy to grade the intestinal metaplasia. Which of the following statements about the oesophagus is true?**

○ A It is about 35 cm long

○ B It mainly occupies the middle mediastinum

○ C It enters the abdomen opposite the twelfth thoracic vertebra

○ D It receives its arterial supply from the thyrocervical trunk

○ E It is supplied by the phrenic nerve

1.55 **A stab wound into the ischiorectal fossa 2 cm lateral to the anal canal is likely to damage:**

○ A The perineal body

○ B The pudendal nerve

○ C The vesicular bulb

○ D The inferior rectal artery

○ E The crus of the penis

1.56 **A 78-year-old man with acute urinary retention was noticed to have benign prostatic hyperplasia on digital examination per rectum. Which of the following statements about the prostate gland is true?**

○ A It is situated immediately above the internal urethral orifice

○ B It is held in place by the ischioprostatic ligaments

○ C It is invested by the inferior fascia of the urogenital diaphragm

○ D It is a purely glandular body

○ E It is perforated by the ejaculatory ducts

anatomy

1.57 **A 17-year-old girl presented in A&E with typical ureteric colic. Which of the following statements about the ureter is true?**

○ A It measures about 15 cm in length

○ B On the right side at its origin it is covered by the ascending part of the duodenum

○ C On the left side it is crossed by the left colic vessels

○ D It receives direct arterial supply from the descending aorta

○ E It is supplied by the genitofemoral nerve

1.58 **A 20-year-old Asian man is seen in the orthopaedics outpatient clinic by a junior house officer with complaints of a large tender mass over the back and a similar mass in the ipsilateral groin. The junior house officer diagnoses tuberculosis of the lumbar spine with a cold abscess that has tracked along a muscle to the groin. Which of the following muscles is most likely to be involved?**

○ A Gluteus maximus

○ B Gluteus minimus

○ C Adductor longus

○ D Psoas major

○ E Piriformis

1.59 **Which of the following statements best describes the transpyloric plane?**

○ A It lies midway between the nipples and the pubic symphysis

○ B It lies roughly a hand's breadth below the xiphisternal joint

○ C It passes anteriorly through the tip of the tenth costal cartilage

○ D It passes posteriorly through the body of the second lumbar vertebra near its lower border

○ E It cuts through the body of the stomach

1.60 **A 25-year-old man arrived in A&E department with a firearm injury to the right popliteal fossa that had severed his popliteal artery. Which of the following statements about the popliteal artery is true?**

○ A It is the continuation of the profunda femoral artery

○ B It divides at the lower border of adductor magnus into its terminal branches

○ C In the middle part of its course, it is crossed from the lateral to the medial side by the tibial nerve and the popliteal vein

○ D It is related laterally to semimembranosus

○ E It is related medially to biceps femoris

1.61 **An acoustic neuroma (tumour of the eighth cranial nerve) is also likely to involve:**

○ A The glossopharyngeal nerve

○ B The abducent nerve

○ C The trigeminal nerve

○ D The facial nerve

○ E The vagus nerve

anatomy

1.62 A bullet entering the right side of the neck at the C4 vertebral level is most likely to injure which of the following structures?

- A   The spinal root of accessory nerve
- B   The superior cervical ganglion
- C   The stellate ganglion
- D   The cricoid cartilage
- E   The bifurcation of common carotid artery

1.63 The movements that take place at the knee joint are flexion and extension and, in certain positions of the joint, internal and external rotation. Which of the following statements about the knee joint is true?

- A   It consists of three articulations in one
- B   It has an anterior cruciate ligament that is stronger and shorter than the posterior cruciate ligament
- C   It has a circular medial meniscus
- D   It has a medial meniscus that covers a larger portion of the articular surface than the lateral one
- E   It has a ligamentum patella that is the central portion of the common tendon of quadratus femoris

1.64 A person is seen in A&E with a shallow knife wound in the posterior triangle of the neck about 1.5 inches (4 cm) above the clavicle. He is complaining of anaesthesia below the wound and over the acromion and clavicle. The nerve most probably injured was:

- A   The greater auricular nerve
- B   The supraclavicular nerve
- C   The lesser occipital nerve
- D   The suprascapular nerve
- E   The transverse cervical nerve

1.65 **Thrombotic occlusion of the coeliac trunk, with preservation of function of the organs supplied by this artery, is possibly caused by anastomosis between:**

○　A　The left gastric artery and right gastric artery

○　B　The left gastroepiploic artery and right gastroepiploic artery

○　C　The proper hepatic artery and gastroduodenal artery

○　D　The right colic artery and middle colic artery

○　E　The superior pancreaticoduodenal artery and inferior pancreaticoduodenal artery

1.66 **Infection from an abscess on the upper eyelid can spread to the dural venous sinuses of the brain as a result of direct communication between the superior ophthalmic vein and:**

○　A　The superior petrosal sinus

○　B　The occipital sinus

○　C　The cavernous sinus

○　D　The sigmoid sinus

○　E　The straight sinus

1.67 **A large benign tumour arising from the choroidal plexus of the lateral ventricle and extending into a surrounding structure is most likely to involve:**

○　A　The pons

○　B　The caudate nucleus

○　C　The cerebellum

○　D　The hippocampus

○　E　The hypothalamus

anatomy

1.68 During clinical examination, a piece of paper is put between adjacent surfaces of the patient's index and middle fingers and he is asked to squeeze them together with sufficient force to hold the paper. This test assesses the function of:

- ○ A The first dorsal and first palmar interosseous muscles
- ○ B The first dorsal and second palmar interosseous muscles
- ○ C The first lumbrical and second dorsal interosseous muscles
- ○ D The second dorsal and first palmar interosseous muscles
- ○ E The second dorsal and second palmar interosseous muscles

1.69 During cholecystectomy accidental injury to a vessel in the area immediately posterior to the epiploic foramen resulted in torrential haemorrhage. The vessel most likely to be involved is:

- ○ A The inferior vena cava
- ○ B The aorta
- ○ C The portal vein
- ○ D The right renal artery
- ○ E The superior mesenteric vein

1.70 During cholecystectomy the cystic artery is usually found in the 'triangle of Calot' formed by:

- ○ A The cystic duct, right hepatic artery and right hepatic duct
- ○ B The gallbladder, liver and common bile duct
- ○ C The left hepatic duct, liver and cystic duct
- ○ D The right branch of the portal vein, liver and common bile duct
- ○ E The common hepatic duct, liver and cystic duct

1.71 The cremasteric muscle is an extension of:

○ A   The external abdominal oblique muscle
○ B   The internal oblique muscle
○ C   The rectus abdominis muscle
○ D   The pyramidalis muscle
○ E   The dartos muscle

1.72 Which of the following structures corresponds to the T8 vertebral level?

○ A   The manubriosternal junction
○ B   The inferior angle of scapula
○ C   The medial end of spine of scapula
○ D   The vena caval opening in diaphragm
○ E   The suprasternal notch

1.73 While mobilising structures in the pelvis to perform abdominoperineal resection, the surgeon accidentally injures a branch of the posterior division of the internal iliac artery. Which of the following is most likely to be injured?

○ A   Superior vesical artery
○ B   Superior gluteal artery
○ C   Obturator artery
○ D   Internal pudendal artery
○ E   Middle rectal artery

anatomy

1.74 The posterior triangle of the neck is bounded by:

○ A The anterior border of the sternocleidomastoid muscle, inferior border of the mandible and anterior midline of the neck

○ B The anterior borders of both sternocleidomastoid muscles, inferior border of the mandible and suprasternal notch of the manubrium

○ C The posterior border of the sternocleidomastoid muscle and clavicle and anterior border of the trapezius muscle

○ D The anterior borders of both trapezius muscles and occipital bone and posterior midline of the neck

○ E Both bellies of the digastric muscle and the inferior border of the mandible

1.75 The phrenic nerve supplies the thoracoabdominal diaphragm. Which of the following statements about the phrenic nerve is true?

○ A It has a root value of C2, C3

○ B It is a pure motor nerve

○ C It runs obliquely across the front of the sternocleidomastoid muscle

○ D It descends almost vertically behind the root of the lung

○ E It is accompanied by the pericardiacophrenic branch of the internal mammary artery in the thorax

1.76 Iatrogenic injury to the thoracodorsal nerve at the time of excision of a lump in the scapular region will affect:

○ A Latissimus dorsi

○ B Serratus anterior

○ C Serratus posterior inferior

○ D Levator scapulae

○ E Longissimus

1.77 **While removing a lump from the sole of the foot the surgeon accidentally injures the medial plantar nerve. Which of the following muscles will be paralysed as a result of this iatrogenic injury?**

- A   Plantar interossei
- B   Second lumbrical
- C   Flexor digitorum brevis
- D   Dorsal Interossei
- E   Abductor digiti minimi

1.78 **The portal vein conveys blood from the abdominal part of the digestive tube (with the exception of the lower part of the rectum) and from the spleen, pancreas and gallbladder to the liver. Which of the following statements about the portal vein is true?**

- A   It is about 20 cm in length
- B   It is formed at the level of the first lumbar vertebra
- C   It is formed by the junction of the inferior mesenteric and splenic veins
- D   It is placed behind and between the common bile duct and the hepatic artery in the lesser omentum
- E   It is surrounded by the portal plexus of nerves

1.79 **Which of the following structures will have intact function after a displaced fracture of the medial epicondyle of humerus?**

- A   Ulnar nerve
- B   Pronator teres
- C   Flexor carpi radialis
- D   Palmaris longus
- E   Flexor digitorum profundus

anatomy

27

anatomy

1.80 A road traffic victim in A&E was noticed to have clinical features suggestive of paralysis of the right suprascapular nerve. Which of the following statements about the suprascapular nerve is true?

○ A It contains nerve fibres from C5 and C6 spinal cord segments

○ B It innervates the teres minor muscle

○ C It provides cutaneous innervation to the posterolateral surface of the shoulder

○ D It is a branch of the middle trunk of the brachial plexus

○ E It courses superior to the suprascapular ligament

1.81 While exposing the internal carotid artery in the carotid triangle for carotid endarterectomy, the surgeon must avoid a vital structure that lies anteromedial to the internal carotid artery. This vital structure is:

○ A The internal jugular vein

○ B The vagus nerve

○ C The external carotid artery

○ D The glossopharyngeal nerve

○ E The hypoglossal nerve

1.82 The pterygoid venous plexus drains the infratemporal fossa via:

○ A The external jugular vein

○ B The internal jugular vein

○ C The posterior auricular vein

○ D The maxillary vein

○ E The superficial temporal vein

anatomy

1.83 **The masseter is an important muscle of mastication. Which of the following statements about the masseter is true?**

- ○ A It extends almost horizontally between the infratemporal fossa and the condyle of the mandible
- ○ B It consists of superficial and deep portions
- ○ C It arises by two heads
- ○ D It assists in opening the mouth
- ○ E It is supplied by the seventh cranial nerve

1.84 **During a carotid endarterectomy, the spinal accessory nerve (cranial nerve XI) is damaged with resultant weakness and atrophy of:**

- ○ A Rhomboid major
- ○ B Teres minor
- ○ C Trapezius
- ○ D Levator scapulae
- ○ E Splenius capitis

1.85 **During cholecystectomy, which of the following gross features of the gallbladder is noticed?**

- ○ A The fundus is completely retroperitoneal
- ○ B The neck is wide and dilated
- ○ C The body is in relation, via its undersurface, with the start of the jejunum
- ○ D The cystic duct of the gallbladder courses independently to the duodenum
- ○ E The fundus of the gallbladder usually lies at the tip of the ninth costal cartilage, in the midclavicular line

1.86 **The Budd–Chiari syndrome is a rare disorder characterised by marked narrowing and occlusion of the hepatic veins resulting in hepatomegaly, ascites and pain in the right upper quadrant of the abdomen. Which of the following statements about the hepatic veins is true?**

○ A They are arranged in two groups

○ B They enter the porta hepatis

○ C In a cross-section of the liver, they are grouped with a hepatic artery and hepatic duct

○ D They drain blood into the portal vein

○ E They contain valves

1.87 **Neurolytic coeliac ganglia block is the therapy of choice for visceral upper abdominal pain that is resistant to therapy. Which of the following statements about the coeliac ganglia is true?**

○ A They are placed on either side of the midline in front of the aorta and vena cava

○ B They are joined by the lesser splanchnic nerves in the upper part

○ C They are parasympathetic ganglia

○ D They are traversed by vagal (parasympathetic) fibres that do not synapse in the ganglia

○ E They receive postganglionic sympathetic fibres from the greater splanchnic nerves

1.88 **An aspiration needle inserted into the ninth intercostal space in the midaxillary line will enter:**

○ A The cupola

○ B The cardiac notch

○ C The oblique pericardial sinus

○ D The costomediastinal recess

○ E The costodiaphragmatic recess

1.89 **While ligating the ductus arteriosus it is important to avoid injury to:**

- ○ A The thoracic duct
- ○ B The left recurrent laryngeal nerve
- ○ C The accessory hemiazygos vein
- ○ D The left internal mammary artery
- ○ E The left phrenic nerve

1.90 **A 50-year-old man presents in an outpatient clinic with a lump in his groin, which on clinical examination was diagnosed as a direct inguinal hernia. His past history suggested that he had undergone an emergency appendicectomy almost 6 months previously. The direct inguinal hernia may well have been caused by iatrogenic injury at the time of appendicectomy to:**

- ○ A The ilioinguinal nerve
- ○ B The subcostal nerve
- ○ C The femoral branch of the genitofemoral nerve
- ○ D The genital branch of the genitofemoral nerve
- ○ E The ventral primary ramus of T10

1.91 **Infection of the mastoid air cells could result from entry of bacteria through:**

- ○ A The sacculus
- ○ B The cochlea
- ○ C The external auditory meatus
- ○ D The internal auditory meatus
- ○ E The nasopharyngeal tube

1.92 **A child was examined by an ENT consultant after iatrogenic rupture of his ear drum. The consultant examined the child for possible injury to a nerve that runs across the eardrum. The most likely nerve to be injured is:**

○ A The glossopharyngeal nerve
○ B The mandibular nerve
○ C The chorda tympani nerve
○ D The lesser petrosal nerve
○ E The great auricular nerve

1.93 **Chemodectoma is a benign tumour of the carotid body. Which of the following statements about the carotid body is true?**

○ A It lies at the termination of the external carotid artery
○ B It is a baroreceptor
○ C It is supplied by the glossopharyngeal nerve
○ D It is similar to the coeliac ganglion
○ E It is a chemoreceptor that monitors serum sodium levels

1.94 **A 45-year-old woman underwent excision of the pisiform bone as a last resort treatment for painful arthritis involving the joint between the pisiform and a neighbouring carpal bone. Which of the following statements about the pisiform bone is true?**

○ A It is situated on a plane posterior to the other carpal bones
○ B It has a single articular facet
○ C It articulates with the trapezoid
○ D It gives attachment to the flexor carpi radialis
○ E It gives attachment to the abductor pollicis brevis

1.95 **Jugular foramen tumours are rare skull-base lesions that present diagnostic and complex management problems. Which of the following statements about the jugular foramen is true?**

○   A   It is situated behind the carotid canal on the base of the skull

○   B   It is divided into two compartments

○   C   It transmits the mandibular nerve

○   D   It transmits the transverse sinus

○   E   It transmits the hypoglossal nerve

1.96 **Which of the following features help to identify the clavicle?**

○   A   It is a short bone

○   B   It has a facet for articulation with the coracoid process of the scapula

○   C   Its medial two-thirds are flattened from above downwards

○   D   The anterior border of the lateral third gives attachment to the deltoid

○   E   The posterior border of the lateral third gives attachment to the sternocleidomastoid

1.97 **The lumbrical muscles of the hand are vital for pianists and typists. Which of the following statements about the lumbrical muscles of the hand is true?**

○   A   There are five in number

○   B   They are associated with the tendons of flexor digitorum superficialis

○   C   They are inserted into the distal interphalangeal joint of the corresponding finger

○   D   They are all innervated by the ulnar nerve

○   E   They assist in extension of the middle and distal phalanges

anatomy

1.98 Twisting of the ankle with forcible eversion during skiing will most probably sprain:

- ○ A The calcaneofibular ligament
- ○ B The anterior talofibular ligament
- ○ C The deltoid ligament
- ○ D The spring ligament
- ○ E The anterior tibiofibular ligament

1.99 The rotator cuff of the shoulder joint will be affected by injury to:

- ○ A Teres major
- ○ B Supraspinatus
- ○ C Latissimus dorsi
- ○ D Pectoralis minor
- ○ E Deltoid

1.100 After a road traffic accident the injured driver is noticed to have injury to an infraclavicular branch of the brachial plexus. The nerve most likely to be involved is:

- ○ A The upper subscapular nerve
- ○ B The suprascapular nerve
- ○ C The dorsal scapular nerve
- ○ D The nerve to subclavius
- ○ E The long thoracic nerve

SECTION 2:
PHYSIOLOGY – QUESTIONS

For each question given below choose the SINGLE BEST option.

2.1 **Insulin is produced by the β cells of the islets of Langerhans in the pancreas. Insulin secretion from endocrine pancreas is inhibited by:**

○ A   Glucagon
○ B α_2-Adrenergic agonists
○ C β_2-Adrenergic agonists
○ D   Cholecystokinin
○ E   Muscarinic agonists

2.2 **Antidiuretic hormone (ADH) is released from the posterior pituitary gland when there is a decrease in plasma:**

○ A   Potassium concentration
○ B   Sodium concentration
○ C   pH
○ D   Volume
○ E   Calcium concentration

2.3 **The second heart sound is produced by the closure of the aortic and pulmonic valves. Closure of the aortic valve occurs at the onset of:**

○ A   The rapid ejection phase of the cardiac cycle
○ B   The isovolumetric contraction phase of the cardiac cycle
○ C   The protodiastole
○ D   The rapid filling phase of the cardiac cycle
○ E   The isovolumetric relaxation phase of the cardiac cycle

2.4 Turbulence in a blood vessel is more likely to occur if:

○ A The velocity of blood within the vessel increases

○ B The diameter of the vessel decreases

○ C The viscosity of blood within the vessel increases

○ D The density of blood decreases

○ E The length of the vessel increases

2.5 The affinity of haemoglobin for oxygen will increase if:

○ A The arterial P_{CO_2} is increased

○ B The pH is decreased

○ C The blood temperature is increased

○ D The H^+ concentration is increased

○ E 2,3-Diphosphoglycerate (DPG) levels in the red blood cells (RBCs) are decreased

2.6 A patient with persistent diarrhoea will have an increased:

○ A Anion gap

○ B Filtered load of bicarbonate

○ C Production of ammonia by the distal tubule

○ D H^+ secretion by the distal tubule

○ E Production of new bicarbonate by the proximal tubule

2.7 **A patient in the A&E department with profuse haemorrhage from a severed limb artery will have increased:**

O   A   Sodium excretion

O   B   Sympathetic nerve activity

O   C   Vagal nerve activity

O   D   Arteriolar diameter in skin

O   E   Water excretion

2.8 **Intestinal peristalsis results in the movement of food through the gut. Intestinal peristalsis:**

O   A   Is controlled by extrinsic innervation

O   B   Is inhibited by vagotomy

O   C   Is inhibited by sympathectomy

O   D   Requires an intact myenteric nerve plexus

O   E   Is inhibited by cholecystokinin

2.9 **Secretin was the first substance that was identified to cause a physiological effect in the body after being transported via the blood. Which of the following statements about secretin is true?**

O   A   It is a polypeptide hormone made up of 17 amino acids

O   B   It increases gallbladder emptying

O   C   It is released by the presence of long-chain fatty acids in the chyme

O   D   It stimulates bicarbonate release from the pancreas

O   E   It inhibits pepsinogen secretion

physiology

2.10 **A 72-year-old woman developed an acute pulmonary embolism 3 days after her total hip replacement. Which of the following features is most likely to be seen in this patient?**

- ○ A Increased P_{CO_2}
- ○ B Increased P_{O_2}
- ○ C Decreased alveolar dead space
- ○ D Decreased right ventricular afterload
- ○ E Increased pulmonary vascular resistance

2.11 **What will be the interstitial osmotic pressure in a skin capillary if fluid is being forced out of it with a net filtration pressure of 8 mmHg when the capillary hydrostatic pressure is 24 mmHg, interstitial hydrostatic pressure 7 mmHg and capillary colloid osmotic pressure 17 mmHg? (Assume that both the filtration coefficient and reflection coefficient in this case are 1.)**

- ○ A 8 mmHg
- ○ B 6 mmHg
- ○ C 9 mmHg
- ○ D −9 mmHg
- ○ E −6 mmHg

physiology

2.12 When air enters the intrapleural space (pneumothorax), the most likely response is for:

○ A The lung to expand outwards and the chest wall to spring inwards

○ B The lung to expand outwards and the chest wall to spring outwards

○ C The lung to collapse inwards and the chest wall to collapse inwards

○ D The lung to collapse inwards and the chest wall to spring outwards

○ E The lung volume to be unaffected and chest wall to spring outwards

2.13 Haemodynamic changes in response to obstruction of venous return to the right side of heart include:

○ A Cardiac output will fall and systemic arterial blood pressure will fall

○ B Cardiac output will rise and systemic arterial blood pressure will rise

○ C Cardiac output will fall and systemic arterial blood pressure will rise

○ D Cardiac output will fall and systemic arterial blood pressure will fall

○ E Cardiac output will remain unchanged and systemic arterial blood pressure will fall

physiology

2.14 Common features of a tumour of the right atrium and cardiac tamponade include:

○　A　Pulmonary oedema, pulmonary hypertension and pulmonary venous congestion

○　B　Pulmonary venous congestion, systemic venous congestion and systemic hypotension

○　C　Systemic oedema, high cardiac output and ascites

○　D　Systemic oedema, congestion of the systemic veins and ascites

○　E　Pulmonary oedema, systemic hypertension and low cardiac output

2.15 Voltage-gated sodium channels are an example of a protein embedded in the plasma membrane of nerve and muscle cells that is used in the rapid electrical signalling found in these cells. Voltage-gated sodium channels:

○　A　Are formed by co-assembly of five identical or similar α subunits

○　B　Have specialised transmembrane domains (S4) that sense transmembrane voltage

○　C　Are equally permeable to K^+ and Na^+

○　D　Are activated by binding of glycine

○　E　Are activated by a decrease in intracellular ATP concentration

2.16 **Cells within the sinoatrial (SA) node are the primary pacemaker site within the heart. These cells are characterised as having no true resting potential, but instead generate regular, spontaneous action potentials. Phase 0 of an SA nodal action potential results from:**

○ A   Activation of sodium channels

○ B   Activation of the pacemaker current

○ C   Influx of Ca^{2+} ions

○ D   Inactivation of K^+ channels

○ E   Influx of Na^+ ions

2.17 **What should the myeloid:erythroid ratio in your bone marrow be if you want to be a voluntary bone marrow donor?**

○ A   1:1

○ B   1:3

○ C   3:1

○ D   1:10

○ E   10:1

2.18 **Substances with high oil:water partition coefficients readily permeate cell membranes. Which group has high oil:water partition coefficients?**

○ A   Peptides, steroid hormones, oxygen

○ B   Steroid hormones, oxygen, ions

○ C   Oxygen, ions, carbon dioxide

○ D   Ions, carbon dioxide, steroid hormones

○ E   Carbon dioxide, steroid hormones, oxygen

physiology

2.19 Stroke volume is the amount of blood pumped by the left ventricle of the heart in one contraction. Which of the following statements about stroke volume is true?

- ○   A   It is the difference between the ventricular end-systolic volume and ventricular end-diastolic volume
- ○   B   It is normally 120 ml in an adult weighing 70 kg
- ○   C   It is decreased by sympathetic activation of the heart
- ○   D   It is increased by increased venous return
- ○   E   It is increased by systemic hypertension

2.20 Which of the following statements about electrolyte concentration of body fluids is correct?

- ○   A   Plasma has 20 mmol/l Mg^{2+}
- ○   B   Interstitial fluid has 10 mmol/l Cl^-
- ○   C   Intracellular fluid has 30 mmol/l HCO_3^-
- ○   D   Plasma has 2.5 mmol/l SO_4^{2-}
- ○   E   Intracellular fluid has 150 mmol/l K^+

2.21 A patient in A&E is noted to have metabolic acidosis with a normal anion gap. Which of the following conditions is most likely to be associated with this abnormality?

- ○   A   Renal failure
- ○   B   Rhabdomyolysis
- ○   C   Lactic acidosis
- ○   D   Alcoholic ketoacidosis
- ○   E   Ureterosigmoidostomy

physiology

2.22 **A patient on the surgical ward is noted to have metabolic alkalosis with a urine Cl⁻ concentration of < 15 mmol/l. Which of the following conditions is most likely to be associated with this abnormality?**

- ○ A Nasogastric suctioning
- ○ B Mineralocorticoid excess
- ○ C Alkali loading
- ○ D Concurrent diuretic administration
- ○ E Severe hypokalaemia

2.23 **The ejection fraction is a measurement of the heart's efficiency and can be used to estimate the function of the left ventricle, which pumps blood to the rest of the body. In a resting healthy individual the ejection fraction is:**

- ○ A 20%
- ○ B 30%
- ○ C 45%
- ○ D > 60%
- ○ E 90%

2.24 **A 42-year-old woman with a small cell carcinoma of her left lung was noticed to have the following biochemical abnormalities: serum sodium 125 mmol/l, plasma osmolality 250 mosmol/kg, inappropriately concentrated urine with osmolality 150 mosmol/kg water and elevated urine sodium concentration 30 mmol/l. Excess of which of the following hormones is responsible for this abnormal biochemical profile?**

- ○ A Thyroxine
- ○ B Oxytocin
- ○ C Cortisol
- ○ D Adrenaline (epinephrine)
- ○ E ADH

physiology

43

2.25 A 65-year-old woman was admitted with an exacerbation of chronic obstructive pulmonary disease. Her arterial blood gases on air showed pH 7.29, $Paco_2$ 8.5 kPa (65.3 mmHg), Pao_2 8.0 kPa (62 mmHg), and standard bicarbonate 30.5 mmol/l. What is the acid–base disturbance?

- ◯ A   Metabolic acidosis
- ◯ B   Respiratory acidosis
- ◯ C   Metabolic alkalosis
- ◯ D   Respiratory alkalosis
- ◯ E   Compensated metabolic acidosis

2.26 The following values were obtained from a Swan–Ganz catheter in a patient who was admitted to an intensive care unit (ICU) with low cardiac output after myocardial infarction:

Cardiac output (CO) = 2.0 l/min

Mean arterial pressure (MAP) = 50 mmHg

Central venous pressure (CVP) = 14 mmHg

Pulmonary artery wedge pressure (PAWP) = 16 mmHg

Mean pulmonary artery pressure (MPAP) = 35 mmHg

What is the systemic vascular resistance in this patient?

- ◯ A   800 dyn/cm^2
- ◯ B   1000 dyn/cm^2
- ◯ C   1440 dyn/cm^2
- ◯ D   1500 dyn/cm^2
- ◯ E   1620 dyn/cm^2

2.27 **A Swan–Ganz catheter inserted into a patient with low cardiac output records a PAWP of 18 mmHg. The same pressure would be expected in which of the following structures?**

- A Systemic veins
- B Right ventricle
- C Left ventricle
- D Aorta
- E Left atrium

2.28 **A 40-year-old man is on injectable vitamin B_{12} replacement therapy after a gastrectomy for a tumour involving the gastric fundus. Absence of which of the following cell types is responsible for this vitamin replacement requirement?**

- A Parietal cells
- B Chief cells
- C G-cells
- D Mucus neck cells
- E Goblet cells

2.29 **Release of ADH from the posterior pituitary gland occurs as a physiological response to a drop in plasma volume or an increase in serum osmolality. In the presence of ADH the glomerular filtrate will be isotonic to plasma in:**

- A The ascending limb of the loop of Henle
- B The cortical collecting tubule
- C The medullary collecting tubule
- D The descending limb of the loop of Henle
- E The renal pelvis

physiology

2.30 A 23-year-old man arrived in A&E in shock with profuse bleeding from his femoral vessels after a gun shot injury to his right groin. Which of the following changes is most likely to be anticipated in this patient?

○   A   Decreased release of thromboxane A_2 at the site of injury

○   B   Increased baseline vagal tone

○   C   Dilatation of veins and venous reservoirs

○   D   Increased renin secretion from the juxtaglomerular apparatus

○   E   Decreased level of circulating ADH

2.31 A 16-year-old girl is admitted with mitral stenosis caused by rheumatic heart disease. A rise in which of the following parameters is consistent with this patient's valvular lesion?

○   A   Aortic pressure

○   B   Cardiac output

○   C   Left atrial pressure

○   D   Left ventricular end-systolic volume

○   E   CVP

2.32 You are looking at an ECG strip that shows sinus bradycardia. Which of the following conditions is most likely to be associated with this ECG finding?

○   A   Hypovolaemia

○   B   Hypothermia

○   C   Vasodilator therapy

○   D   Injection of atropine

○   E   Fever

2.33 A 48-year-old woman presents to her doctor complaining of weakness and fatigue. On physical examination, her weight is up by 10 pounds (4.5 kg) compared with her last visit 6 months ago. Her blood pressure (BP) is 160/100 mmHg. Blood tests reveal serum Na$^+$ 155 mmol/l, K$^+$ 2..8 mmol/l and a decreased serum renin. Which of the following is the most likely diagnosis?

○ A   Cushing's syndrome

○ B   Diabetes mellitus

○ C   Phaeochromocytoma

○ D   Primary aldosteronism

○ E   Secondary aldosteronism

2.34 A patient is given an intravenous infusion of *p*-aminohippuric acid (PAH). After a short time, the plasma PAH is 0.02 mg/ml, concentration of PAH in urine 13 mg/ml and urine flow 1.0 ml/min. What is the effective renal plasma flow?

○ A   0.26 ml/min

○ B   26 ml/min

○ C   65 ml/min

○ D   260 ml/min

○ E   650 ml/min

2.35 A 45-year-old obese woman experiences episodic abdominal pain. She notes that the pain increases after the ingestion of a fatty meal. The action of which of the following hormones is responsible for the postprandial intensification of her symptoms?

○ A   Cholecystokinin

○ B   Gastrin

○ C   Pepsin

○ D   Secretin

○ E   Somatostatin

physiology

2.36 Bile is a complex fluid containing water, electrolytes, and a battery of organic molecules including bile acids, cholesterol, phospholipids and bilirubin, which flows through the biliary tract into the small intestine. Which of the following statements about bile is true?

○ A Adult humans produce about 150–200 ml of bile daily

○ B Bile acids are derivatives of cholesterol synthesised in the hepatocytes

○ C Hepatocytes add bicarbonate to the bile

○ D Bile salts are purely hydrophobic

○ E Of the bile acids delivered to the duodenum 5% are absorbed back into the blood within the ileum

2.37 A 25-year-old man has cholecystokinin deficiency as a component of an autoimmune polyglandular syndrome. Which of the following effects is likely to be seen in this patient as a result of cholecystokinin deficiency?

○ A Increased pancreatic enzyme secretion

○ B Enhanced gallbladder contraction

○ C Contraction of the sphincter of Oddi

○ D Inhibition of gastric emptying

○ E Stimulation of small bowel motility

2.38 **A 55-year-old man with gradual onset of weight loss, diarrhoea, stomatitis and a necrolytic migrating erythema develops diabetes mellitus. On investigation he is diagnosed as having a tumour of the α cells of pancreas. Which of the following physiological abnormalities is most likely to be present in this patient?**

○   A   Inhibition of gluconeogenesis
○   B   Inhibition of lipolysis
○   C   Inhibition of catecholamine secretion
○   D   Activation of glycogenolysis
○   E   Stimulation of gastric secreting activity

2.39 **A 46-year-old man with a mechanical mitral valve and atrial fibrillation developed mesenteric ischaemia as a result of thromboembolism from the valve. Upon exploratory laparotomy the whole of the jejunum was noticed to be gangrenous and resected. Absorption of which of the following substances is likely to be affected in this patient?**

○   A   Vitamin B_{12}
○   B   Water
○   C   Electrolytes
○   D   Bile salts
○   E   Fat-soluble vitamins

physiology

2.40 After a total hip replacement a 78-year-old woman developed a pulmonary embolism that caused obstruction of a branch of the pulmonary artery. Which of the following is likely to increase in this patient?

○ A Ventilation/perfusion ratio

○ B Lung volume

○ C Arterial CO_2

○ D Arterial O_2

○ E Alveolar O_2 saturation

2.41 A woman pulled from a fire is markedly hypoxic. Respiration in this patient will be rapidly influenced by hypoxia through its stimulatory effect:

○ A Directly on the medullary respiratory neurons

○ B Directly on the pulmonary mechanoreceptors

○ C On the central chemoreceptors

○ D On the carotid and aortic chemoreceptors

○ E Directly on the $Hb-O_2$ dissociation curve

2.42 A 66-year-old man who is a chronic smoker is admitted for elective repair of a right-sided indirect inguinal hernia. His clinical examination and chest radiological findings are consistent with chronic obstructive airway disease. He is sent for pulmonary function tests. Which of the following abnormalities is most likely to be present in this patient?

○ A Increased FEV_1/FVC (forced expiratory volume in 1 s/forced vital capacity)

○ B Decreased total lung capacity (TLC)

○ C Increased residual volume (RV)

○ D Decreased functional residual capacity (FRC)

○ E Increased carbon monoxide diffusing capacity ($DLCO$)

2.43 **A patient with deteriorating renal function is to undergo estimation of his glomerular filtration rate (GFR). Which of the following substances will be the best choice for the estimation of GFR in this patient?**

○ A Urea

○ B Inulin

○ C PAH

○ D Creatinine

○ E ^{51}Cr-labelled EDTA

2.44 **A 76-year-old woman undergoes a sigmoid colectomy for a ruptured diverticulum. Her baseline blood pressure is 140/80 mmHg. She requires multiple boluses of phenylephrine in the operating room to support her blood pressure. On return to intensive care, the patient is mechanically ventilated and her blood pressure is 90/50 mmHg. Her urinary output is 15 ml in the first hour. Which of the following is the best strategy to improve her urine output?**

○ A Start infusion of an inotrope

○ B Give intravenous corticosteroids

○ C Insert a Swan–Ganz catheter

○ D Use a stroke volume monitor

○ E Fluid challenge followed by vasopressor

physiology

2.45 A 65-year-old man with a history of hypertension (usual BP 150/90) and intermittent atrial fibrillation is admitted in A&E with a 6-hour history of a painful white leg. A large embolus is located in his left internal iliac artery, with distal ischaemia. He is brought to the operating room for embolectomy–revascularisation. Just before induction his BP is 200/100 mmHg, which is treated with a labetalol infusion. Once circulation to the affected limb is re-established successfully, the BP falls to 160/90 mmHg and the labetalol infusion is stopped. The patient is otherwise stable and is returned to the ICU postoperatively. Preoperatively his creatinine was 1.1 mg/dl; 6 h postoperatively it was 1.8 mg/dl. His urine was noticed to be tea coloured. The next morning the patient becomes anuric with a creatinine of 2.5 mg/dl. His potassium is 6.8 mmol/l and phosphate 5.9 mg/dl. There is no evidence of postrenal obstruction. He is started on continuous haemofiltration. Which of the following is the most likely cause for this patient's acute renal failure?

○ A   Systemic hypertension

○ B   Labetalol infusion

○ C   Rhabdomyolyis

○ D   Hyperkalaemia

○ E   Atrial fibrillation

2.46 **A 26-year-old man falls from a ladder and sustains injury to the back of his neck. Computed tomography (CT) reveals a bony fragment that penetrated the lateral portion of the dorsal columns. Which of the following functions is most likely to be affected by this lesion?**

- ○ A Vibratory sensations from the ipsilateral arm
- ○ B Fine motor control of the ipsilateral fingers
- ○ C Motor control of the contralateral foot
- ○ D Sweating of the ipsilateral face
- ○ E Proprioception from the ipsilateral leg

2.47 **A 55-year-old man is admitted to an ICU with acute respiratory distress syndrome. Which of the following variables is most likely to be lower than normal in this patient?**

- ○ A Oncotic pressure of alveolar fluid
- ○ B Work of breathing
- ○ C Lung compliance
- ○ D Alveolar–arterial pressure difference
- ○ E Surface tension of alveolar fluid

2.48 **A 43-year-old man has a parathyroid adenoma producing elevated levels of parathyroid hormone. Which of the following statements about parathyroid hormone is true?**

- ○ A Increased ionised calcium levels are essential for its release
- ○ B It causes increased deposition of calcium in bones
- ○ C It stimulates production of the active form of vitamin D in the small intestine
- ○ D It stimulates loss of phosphate ions in the urine
- ○ E It stimulates excretion of calcium in the urine

physiology

2.49 Hypoxia generally causes vasodilatation in arterial beds. In which organ does hypoxia cause vasoconstriction of arterial beds?

○ A Skeletal muscle

○ B Heart

○ C Kidney

○ D Gut

○ E Lungs

2.50 Tissue plasminogen activator (tPA) is a naturally occurring thrombolytic substance. The thrombolytic mechanism of action of tPA involves:

○ A Proteolytic breakdown of fibrin

○ B Direct conversion of plasminogen to plasmin

○ C Depletion of α_2-antiplasmin

○ D Proteolytic activation of fibrinogen

○ E Formation of an active complex with plasminogen

2.51 The liver function tests of a patient show hyperbilirubinaemia. The bilirubin is predominantly conjugated. Which of the following conditions is most likely to be associated with an increase in conjugated bilirubin?

○ A Physiological jaundice of the newborn

○ B Haemolysis caused by rhesus incompatibility

○ C Acute haemolytic crisis in sickle cell disease

○ D Obstructive jaundice resulting from carcinoma of the head of the pancreas

○ E Gilbert's syndrome

2.52 A 22-year-old man with aortic stenosis caused by a congenital bicuspid valve is to undergo aortic valve replacement. On preoperative assessment the oxygen consumption in this patient is 300 ml/min, arterial O_2 content 20 ml/100 ml blood, pulmonary arterial oxygen content 15 ml/100 ml blood and his heart rate 100 beats/min. What is the cardiac stroke volume in this patient?

- A 1 ml
- B 10 ml
- C 60 ml
- D 100 ml
- E 200 ml

2.53 A patient with a ruptured spleen and fractured pelvis as a result of a road traffic accident arrives in A&E in a state of shock. Which of the following organs with the largest specific blood flow per gram of tissue under resting conditions is most vulnerable in this patient?

- A Kidney
- B Heart
- C Brain
- D Skin
- E Skeletal muscle

physiology

2.54 **A 13-year-old boy is diagnosed with a growth hormone (GH)-secreting tumour of the anterior pituitary gland. Which of the following metabolic effects resulting from increased GH secretion is most likely to be enhanced in this patient?**

- ○ A Decreased amino acid uptake
- ○ B Enhanced oxidation of proteins
- ○ C Enhanced triglyceride synthesis
- ○ D Decreased fat oxidation in adipocytes
- ○ E Enhanced glucose synthesis in the liver

2.55 **A steel furnace worker is admitted in A&E with severe acute dehydration. This patient is most likely to have:**

- ○ A High renal water excretion
- ○ B Low permeability of collecting duct tubular cells for water
- ○ C Low plasma ADH levels
- ○ D Decreased baroreceptor firing rate
- ○ E Decreased plasma osmolality

2.56 **Omeprazole is an acid-activated prodrug that binds covalently to the proton pump located at the apical membrane of the gastric parietal cells, resulting in its irreversible inactivation. Which of the following is the site of action of omeprazole?**

- ○ A Active H^+ and Cl^- co-transport
- ○ B H^+/K^+ ATPase
- ○ C Cl^-/HCO_3^- exchange
- ○ D Passive diffusion of H^+
- ○ E Na^+/K^+ pump

2.57 **When a patient has a lower than normal haemoglobin, it is important to determine whether RBCs are of normal size and whether they have a normal concentration of Hb. These measurements, known as erythrocyte or RBC indices, provide important information about various types of anaemia. Which of the following is correct?**

- A   Mean corpuscular volume (MCV) = Haematocrit x Total RBC count
- B   MCV = Hb x Total RBC count
- Ć   Mean corpuscular haemoglobin (MCH) = Haemoglobin x [Total RBC count/100]
- D   MCH concentration (MCHC) = [Haemoglobin/Haematocrit] x 100
- E   MCHC = Haemoglobin/Total RBC count

2.58 **A 22-year-old woman with paroxysmal hypertension, tachycardia, diaphoresis, tachypnoea, flushing, cold and clammy skin, severe headache, angina and palpitation is diagnosed with a phaeochromocytoma. The urine levels of which of the following substances will be high in this patient?**

- A   Dehydroepiandrosterone
- B   Pregnanetriol
- C   Cortisol
- D   Homovanillic acid
- E   5-Hydroxyindoleacetic acid

physiology

2.59 **Multiple endocrine neoplasia (MEN) is a group of genetically distinct familial diseases involving adenomatous hyperplasia and malignant tumour formation in several endocrine glands. Which of the following statements about MEN is true?**

○ A MEN 1 is characterised by tumours of the parathyroid gland, pancreatic islet cells and pituitary gland

○ B MEN 1 is characterised by medullary carcinoma of the thyroid, phaeochromocytoma and hyperparathyroidism

○ C MEN 2A is characterised by multiple mucosal neuroma, medullary carcinoma of the thyroid and phaeochromocytoma, often associated with a marfanoid habitus

○ D MEN 2A is characterised by tumours of pancreatic islet cells and panhypopituitarism

○ E MEN 2B is characterised by tumours of the parathyroid glands, pancreatic islet cells and pituitary gland

2.60 **Calcium is required for the proper functioning of numerous intracellular and extracellular processes, including muscle contraction, nerve conduction, hormone release and blood coagulation. Which of the following conditions is associated with hypocalcaemia?**

○ A Vitamin D excess
○ B Magnesium depletion
○ C Sarcoidosis
○ D Immobilisation
○ E Milk-alkali syndrome

2.61 Magnesium is the fourth most plentiful cation in the body. Which of the following statements about magnesium metabolism is true?

○ A   A 70-kg adult has roughly 200 mmol magnesium

○ B   The extracellular fluid contains about 50% total body magnesium

○ C   Normal plasma magnesium concentration ranges from 0.70 to 1.05 mmol/l (1.4 to 2.1 mequiv/l)

○ D   About 10% of plasma magnesium is ultrafiltered by the kidneys

○ E   Magnesium is the key electrolyte for generation of a smooth muscle action potential

2.62 The parasympathetic nervous system (PNS) is a subdivision of the autonomic nervous system, and it operates in tandem with the other subdivision, the sympathetic nervous system. Which of the following is an effect of stimulation of the PNS?

○ A   Dilatation of the pupils

○ B   Decreased secretion of the lacrimal glands

○ C   Bronchodilatation

○ D   Bradycardia

○ E   Ejaculation

2.63 After cardiac surgery a patient has a very fast heart rate. The ECG of this patient will show:

○ A   A wider QRS complex

○ B   A prolonged P–R interval

○ C   A smaller QRS complex

○ D   A longer ST segment

○ E   A shortened Q–T interval

physiology

2.64 **Atrial fibrillation occurs when the atria depolarise repeatedly and in an irregular uncontrolled manner, usually at an atrial rate greater than 350 beats/min. No P waves are observed in the ECG as a result of the chaotic atrial depolarisation. Which of the following statements about P waves is true?**

○ A The P-wave duration is normally < 0.12 s

○ B The P-wave amplitude is normally > 0.25 mV

○ C The P-wave contour is usually saw-toothed

○ D A negative P wave can indicate depolarisation arising from the bundle of His

○ E The P–R interval is the time (in seconds) from the beginning of the P wave to the end of the QRS complex

2.65 **A 63-year-old man with severe epigastric pain and raised troponin I levels has ECG changes that suggest an acute myocardial infarction involving the inferior wall of the heart. Which of the following ECG leads will pick up these changes?**

○ A V1–V3

○ B II, III, aVF

○ C RV4, RV5

○ D I, aVL, V4–V6

○ E V1–V6

physiology

2.66 **Potassium affects the way the cell membranes work and governs the action of the heart and the pathways between the brain and the muscles. Which of the following statements about potassium metabolism is true?**

◯   A   98% of potassium is extracellular

◯   B   Total body potassium stores are approximately 100 mmol/kg (7000 mmol in a 70-kg person)

◯   C   The liver determines potassium homeostasis

◯   D   Early changes of hyperkalaemia include inverted T waves and a prolonged Q–T interval

◯   E   Acidosis results in hyperkalaemia

2.67 **A phospholipase is an enzyme that converts phospholipids into fatty acids and other lipophilic substances. There are four major classes, termed A, B, C and D. Phospholipase C acts as a secondary messenger. Which of the following statements about phospholipase C is true?**

◯   A   It frees a fatty acid bound in an ester linkage to carbon–2 of glycerol

◯   B   Its activity is stimulated by hormone–receptor interactions coupled to a Gp protein

◯   C   It initiates a cascade, resulting in the activation of protein kinase A

◯   D   It initiates a cascade, resulting in the activation of guanylyl kinase

◯   E   It initiates a cascade, resulting in the activation of tyrosine kinase

physiology

2.68 Oedema is defined as an abnormal accumulation of fluid in tissues or cavities of the body. Oedema may be mechanical – the result of obstructed veins or heart failure – or caused by increased permeability of the capillary walls, as in liver or kidney disease or malnutrition. In the table below which of the physiological derangements will result in pitting oedema and a decrease in plasma osmolality?

		Gain/Loss	Total body fluid	Total body sodium
O	A	Loss	Marked decrease	Decrease
O	B	Gain	Marked increase	Increase
O	C	Gain	Increase	Increase
O	D	Gain	Increase	Marked increase
O	E	Loss	Decrease	Marked decrease

2.69 The total body sodium content is regulated by a balance between dietary intake and renal excretion. Which of the following statements about sodium metabolism is true?

O A Sodium concentration is highest in the intracellular fluid

O B Active transport of sodium across all cells consumes most of the energy derived from cellular metabolism

O C Sodium reabsorption across proximal tubular cells is mainly active and transcellular

O D Sodium concentration gradient provides energy for the co-transport of H^+

O E Transport of sodium across the apical membrane of the nephron is an active transport process

2.70 **The evaluation of the jugular venous pulse (JVP) is an integral part of the physical examination because it reflects both the mean right atrial pressure and the haemodynamic events in the right atrium. Which of the following statements about the JVP waveform is true?**

○   A   The 'a' wave is caused by right ventricular contraction

○   B   The 'c' wave is the most prominent during inspiration

○   C   The 'x' descent results from the increase in blood volume in the vena cavae and the right atrium during ventricular systole when the tricuspid valve is closed

○   D   The 'v' wave is a result of the downward displacement of the tricuspid valve during right ventricular systole

○   E   The 'y' descent is caused by opening of the tricuspid valve

2.71 **In the normal JVP waveform there are three positive waves and two negative troughs. Which of the following statements about abnormalities of these waves and troughs is true?**

○   A   The 'a' wave in the JVP is absent in sinus bradycardia

○   B   Cannon 'a' waves are seen in tricuspid regurgitation

○   C   The 'cv' wave is a feature of tricuspid stenosis

○   D   The 'v' wave is equal to the 'a' wave in patients with an atrial septal defect

○   E   A sharp 'y' descent is a feature of left-sided heart failure

physiology

2.72 Ketoacidosis is a type of metabolic acidosis that is caused by high concentrations of keto acids, formed by the deamination of amino acids. Which of the following conditions is associated with ketoacidosis?

○   A   Expanded blood volume
○   B   Increased lipid synthesis
○   C   Positive nitrogen balance
○   D   Type 2 diabetes
○   E   Low plasma C-peptide levels

2.73 Vasoconstrictors are used clinically to increase BP or to reduce local blood flow. Which of the following naturally occurring peptides produces intense vasoconstriction?

○   A   Neurotensin
○   B   Atrial natriuretic peptide
○   C   Endothelin
○   D   Bradykinin
○   E   Substance P

2.74 A patient has an immunological tubulointerstitial disease process that has destroyed the juxtaglomerular apparatus in his kidneys. Which of the following abnormalities will be seen in this patient?

○   A   Hyperaldosteronism
○   B   Hyperkalaemia
○   C   Increase in angiotensin II
○   D   Metabolic alkalosis
○   E   Loss of H^+ in the urine

2.75 After coronary artery bypass surgery a 56-year-old man develops atelectasis of both lung bases. The physiotherapist advises him that deep inspiration followed by gradual expiration will be good for him. Which of the following events takes place during deep inspiration?

○   A   The pressure gradient between the peripheral veins and the right atrium decreases

○   B   Pulmonary blood volume decreases

○   C   Cardiac output of the right ventricle increases

○   D   Cardiac output of the left ventricle increases

○   E   Venous return to the left atrium increases

2.76 A patient with low systemic vascular resistance after cardiac surgery is started on an infusion of a vasoconstrictor agent. Which of the following effects is likely to be produced by the vasoconstrictor agent in this patient?

○   A   Increased end-diastolic volume

○   B   Decreased preload

○   C   Decreased stroke volume

○   D   Increased end-diastolic reserve volume

○   E   Decreased work of the heart

physiology

2.77 γ motor neurons regulate the sensitivity of the muscle spindle to muscle stretching. With activation of γ neurons, intrafusal muscle fibres contract so that only a small stretch is required to activate spindle sensory neurons and the stretch reflex. Which of the following statements about the γ motor neurons is correct?

○ A   They are inhibited by Golgi tendon organs

○ B   They are inhibited by descending motor tracts

○ C   They are stimulated by 1a afferents

○ D   They are inhibited by 1a afferents

○ E   They are located in the posterior horn of the spinal cord

2.78 The transmembrane voltage changes that take place during an action potential result from changes in the permeability of the membrane to specific ions; the internal and external concentrations of these are maintained in an imbalance by the cells. Minimally, an action potential involves a depolarisation, a repolarisation and finally a hyperpolarisation. The repolarisation phase of an action potential is a result of:

○ A   Increasing activity of the Na^+/K^+ pump

○ B   Increasing Na^+ permeability and increasing K^+ permeability

○ C   Increasing Na^+ permeability and decreasing K^+ permeability

○ D   Decreasing Na^+ permeability and rapidly increasing K^+ permeability

○ E   Decreasing Na^+ permeability and a delayed increasing K^+ permeability

2.79 Calcium is the so-called 'trigger' for muscle contraction. In the skeletal muscle calcium initiates contraction by:

○ A   Being released from the sarcolemma during an action potential

○ B   Binding to tropomyosin

○ C   Binding to troponin

○ D   Covering actin-binding sites

○ E   Binding to myosin cross-bridges

2.80 The human retina has on-centre cells and off-centre cells that are distinguished by the way in which they respond to light on the centres of their receptive fields. In response to light on the retina, the major difference between on-centre cells and off-centre cells is:

○ A   Bipolar cells in on centres depolarise and the bipolar cells in off centres hyperpolarise in response to light

○ B   Bipolar cells in on centres hyperpolarise and the bipolar cells in off centres depolarise in response to light

○ C   Ganglion cells in on centres hyperpolarise and the ganglion cells in off centres depolarise in response to light

○ D   Rods stimulate on centres whereas cones stimulate off centres

○ E   Rods stimulate off centres whereas cones stimulate on centres

physiology

2.81 A 75-year-old woman who has difficulty understanding conversation, particularly when background noise is present, and complains that others mumble is diagnosed as having presbycusis. Which of the following is the most likely to occur in this disorder?

○ A Nystagmus

○ B Loss of sensitivity to angular acceleration

○ C Loss of sensitivity to linear acceleration

○ D Loss of sensitivity to high-frequency sounds

○ E Loss of sensitivity to low-frequency sounds

2.82 Skeletal muscle fibres can be divided into two basic types: type I (slow-twitch fibres) and type II (fast-twitch fibres). Which of the following statements best distinguishes type II from type I muscle fibres?

○ A Type II muscle fibres are rich in mitochondria

○ B Type II muscle fibres are rich in glycogen

○ C Type II muscle fibres function best in aerobic exercise conditions

○ D Type II muscle fibres are the dominant fibres in the postural muscles

○ E Type II fibres do not hypertrophy with exercise

2.83 A 65-year-old man developed spasticity secondary to an upper motor neuron lesion caused by a stroke. Which of the following is most likely to be found in the muscles of this patient?

○ A Increased muscle tone

○ B Atrophy

○ C Paraesthesia

○ D Fasciculations

○ E Less active stretch reflexes

physiology

2.84 **A marathon runner was disqualified from the Athens Olympics because he was found to have used erythropoietin to enhance endurance. Which of the following features is a marker of erythropoietin-stimulated bone marrow?**

○ A Low reticulocyte count

○ B Decreased radioactive plasma iron turnover

○ C Decreased serum ferritin

○ D Increased myeloid:erythroid ratio

○ E Shift cells in the peripheral blood film

2.85 **The blood clotting system or coagulation pathway, similar to the complement system, is a proteolytic cascade. Which of the following statements about the coagulation pathway is true?**

○ A The Hagemann factor (factor XII), factor XI, prekallikrein and high-molecular-weight kininogen are involved in the extrinsic pathway of coagulation

○ B The intrinsic pathway provides a very rapid response to tissue injury, generating activated factor X almost instantaneously

○ C The intrinsic and extrinsic systems converge at factor X to a single common pathway, which is ultimately responsible for the production of thrombin (factor IIa)

○ D The end result of the clotting pathway is the production of fibrin for the conversion of prothrombin to thrombin

○ E The coagulation pathway acts independently of other plasma enzyme systems

physiology

2.86 A 45-year-old woman has an infarct affecting the cerebellum. Which of the following movement defects is she most likely to develop?

○ A Chorea

○ B Athetosis

○ C Resting tremor

○ D Intention tremor

○ E Tics

2.87 A 65-year-old man has developed obstructive jaundice as a result of a carcinoma of the head of the pancreas obstructing the common bile duct. Which of the following biochemical abnormalities will be seen in this patient?

○ A Decreased bilirubin in the urine

○ B Decreased urobilinogen in the stool

○ C Increased urobilinogen in the urine

○ D Decreased plasma direct bilirubin

○ E Decreased plasma conjugated bilirubin

2.88 Scattered throughout the exocrine tissue of the pancreas are several hundred thousand clusters of endocrine cells that produce the hormones insulin and glucagon, plus a few other hormones. Which of the following features do both insulin and glucagon have in common?

○ A Both increase hepatic gluconeogenesis

○ B Both increase hepatic glycogenolysis

○ C Both increase the activity of hormone-sensitive lipase

○ D The secretion of both is increased by hypoglycaemia

○ E The secretion of both is increased by amino acids in the blood

2.89 Urine specific gravity measures the concentration of particles in the urine. The normal specific gravity ranges between 1.005 and 1.030. A urine specific gravity that remains the same when measured during the day or night indicates:

○ A   Loss of concentrating and diluting capacity

○ B   Prerenal azotaemia

○ C   A reduction in the solute load

○ D   Intact tubular function

○ E   Acute glomerular disease

2.90 Five days after coronary artery bypass surgery a patient developed hyperkalaemia as a result of taking a potassium supplement and spironolactone. Which of the following therapies will be ineffective in treating hyperkalaemia in this patient?

○ A   Intravenous insulin and glucose

○ B   Intravenous calcium chloride

○ C   Sodium polystyrene sulphonate enema

○ D   Oral enalapril

○ E   Haemodialysis

2.91 A 22-year-old woman developed a pleural effusion. It was drained and a sample of pleural fluid was sent to the laboratory for analysis. Which of the following statements about the pleural fluid is true?

○ A   The normal volume of pleural fluid is 125 ml

○ B   It has an acidic pH

○ C   The pleural fluid glucose content is the same as the plasma glucose content

○ D   The normal protein content is > 40 g/l

○ E   The normal pleural fluid has no cells

physiology

2.92 A 26-year-old motorcyclist arrived in A&E after an accident. He was conscious and haemodynamically stable. The only significant finding was leakage of clear fluid from the nose. To confirm the diagnosis of cerebrospinal fluid (CSF) rhinorrhoea a sample of the fluid was sent for immunoelectrophoresis. Which of the following statements about CSF is true?

○   A   The normal circulating volume of CSF is 500 ml

○   B   Circulating CSF is absorbed into the lymphatic circulation through the cranial arachnoid granulations and spinal arachnoid villi

○   C   Normal CSF pressure is 100–200 mmHg

○   D   The normal CSF protein content is 20–45 mg/l

○   E   The normal CSF glucose range is 50–100 mg/dl

2.93 A 45-year-old woman developed position-sensitive vertigo accompanied by nausea, vomiting and malaise after a recent viral illness. She was told that she had an inflammation or dysfunction of the vestibular labyrinth, which would resolve after a few days. Which of the following statements about the vestibular labyrinth is true?

○   A   The vestibular labyrinth consists of the cochlea and otolith organs

○   B   The utricle senses motion in the horizontal plane

○   C   The semicircular canals are sensitive to motion in the sagittal plane

○   D   The sensory portion of the otolith organs is the ampulla

○   E   The structure of the utricle and saccule is similar to that of the semicircular canals

physiology

2.94 The neurological examination of a 63-year-old patient with diabetes reveals a lesion involving the right anterior spinothalamic tract at the level of the sixth cervical vertebra. The patient will have:

○ A Contralateral loss of crude touch and pressure sensation below the level of the lesion

○ B Contralateral loss of pain and temperature sensation below the level of the lesion

○ C Ipsilateral loss of crude touch and pressure sensation below the level of the lesion

○ D Ipsilateral loss of pain and temperature sensation below the level of the lesion

○ E Loss of the ability consciously to perceive the position and movements of the ipsilateral limb below the level of the lesion

2.95 The liver receives a dual blood supply. Which of the following statements about hepatic circulation is true?

○ A The portal area can hold about three-quarters of the total blood volume

○ B The average minute blood flow in the hepatic circulation is about 300 ml/100 g of liver tissue

○ C The hepatic artery supplies 50% of the total hepatic blood flow

○ D Pressure in the portal vein is about 8–10 mmHg

○ E Hepatic blood flow increases during moderate exercise

physiology

2.96 A 65-year-old man had an embolic stroke that affected his dominant Broca's area. This patient will have:

○ A Sensory aphasia

○ B Anomic aphasia

○ C Receptive aphasia

○ D Global aphasia

○ E Motor aphasia

2.97 A 78-year-old man with urinary hesitancy and orthostatic hypotension is seen in A&E. On clinical examination he had pill-rolling movements of his right hand, bradykinesia and rest tremor. The patient most probably has a lesion involving:

○ A The motor cortex

○ B The neostriatum

○ C The substantia nigra

○ D The hypothalamus

○ E The red nucleus

2.98 A weightlifter was banned from competing in international events after unusually high levels of testosterone were detected in his blood during random dope testing at the Commonwealth Games. Which of the following statements about testosterone is true?

○ A It binds to the cell surface receptor

○ B It is reduced to dehydroepiandrosterone by the cytoplasmic enzyme 5α-reductase

○ C It decreases bone density

○ D It stimulates bone marrow

○ E It has no effect on the larynx

2.99 **Immunoglobulins are glycoproteins in the immunoglobulin superfamily that function as antibodies. They are grouped into five classes or isotypes: IgG, IgA, IgM, IgD and IgE. Which of the following statements about Ig isotypes is true?**

○ A IgG is the most abundant immunoglobulin
○ B IgA is the only isotype that can pass through placenta
○ C IgM has the smallest molecular mass
○ D IgD mainly acts as opsonin
○ E IgE is a polymeric immunoglobulin

2.100 **Serial lactate determinations may be helpful in patients resuscitated from shock to assess the adequacy of therapies. Which of the following statements about lactate is true?**

○ A The normal blood lactate concentration in unstressed patients is 2.5–3.5 mmol/l
○ B The Cori cycle deals with conversion of glucose to lactate and vice versa
○ C Lactate turnover in healthy resting humans is approximately 130 mmol every 24 hours
○ D Lactate producers are the liver, kidneys and heart
○ E Lactate is a by-product of glycogenolysis

physiology

SECTION 3:
PATHOLOGY – QUESTIONS

For each question given below choose the SINGLE BEST option.

3.1 Bronchial biopsy of a 58-year-old man who is a chronic smoker showed squamous metaplasia. Which of the following statements best describes metaplasia?

○   A   It is an irreversible change
○   B   It is an adaptive response
○   C   It occurs only in epithelium
○   D   It is characterised by cloudy swelling of cells
○   E   It results from a change in the phenotype of a differentiated cell type

3.2 A 60-year-old woman with a long history of poorly controlled type 2 diabetes mellitus has had extensive black discoloration of the skin and soft tissue of her right foot and calf, with areas of yellowish exudate, for the past month. A mixed growth of aerobes and anaerobes is cultured from this exudate. A below-knee amputation is performed. The amputation specimen sent to the histopathology laboratory is most likely to demonstrate which of the following pathological abnormalities?

○   A   Neoplasia
○   B   Coagulopathy
○   C   Haemosiderosis
○   D   Caseation necrosis
○   E   Gangrenous necrosis

pathology

77

3.3 **A 22-year-old man who is a motorcyclist is involved in a high-impact road traffic accident on the motorway which results in multiple blunt trauma and lacerations to his lower extremities. The left femoral artery is lacerated, and he incurs extensive blood loss and remains hypotensive for hours during transport to the accident and emergency department (A&E). On admission, his haematocrit is 15%. Which of the following tissues is most likely to sustain the least damage as a result of prolonged hypotension?**

○ A Small intestinal epithelium
○ B Skeletal muscle
○ C Retina
○ D Myocardium
○ E Hippocampus

3.4 **A histopathology report mentioned the term 'fat necrosis'. Fat necrosis is a feature of:**

○ A Brain injury
○ B Muscle injury
○ C Trauma to the bowel
○ D Acute pancreatitis
○ E Trauma to the uterus

3.5 **A fair-skinned child develops sunburn within 24 hours of exposure to sun. This is caused by:**

○ A Free radical injury
○ B Ischaemic injury
○ C Direct endothelial injury
○ D Chemical injury
○ E Hypoxic injury

pathology

3.6 **Report of a biopsy specimen sent to the histopathology laboratory came back claiming 'no granuloma seen'. The patient is most likely to have which of the following conditions?**

○ A Lepromatous leprosy
○ B Tuberculosis (TB)
○ C Coccidioidomycosis
○ D Syphilis
○ E Trypanosomiasis

3.7 **A patient with an inflammatory condition was told by the consultant that he has features consistent with a type II hypersensitivity reaction. This patient is most likely to have which of the following disorders?**

○ A Polyarteritis nodosa
○ B Reactive arthritis
○ C Serum sickness
○ D Graves' disease
○ E Arthus reaction

3.8 **On receiving intravenous penicillin, a child develops urticaria, dyspnoea and generalised oedema immediately as a result of:**

○ A Type I hypersensitivity
○ B Type II hypersensitivity
○ C Type III hypersensitivity
○ D Type IV hypersensitivity
○ E Systemic immune complex disease

pathology

3.9 **A 50-year-old marketing executive has complained of mild burning epigastric pain after meals for the past 3 years. Upper gastrointestinal (GI) endoscopy is performed and biopsies are taken of an erythematous area of the lower oesophageal mucosa 3 cm above the gastro-oesophageal junction. There is no mass lesion, no ulceration and no haemorrhage noted. The biopsies demonstrate the presence of columnar epithelium with goblet cells. Which of the following mucosal alterations is most probably represented by these findings?**

- ○ A Metaplasia
- ○ B Dysplasia
- ○ C Hyperplasia
- ○ D Carcinoma
- ○ E Ischaemia

3.10 **A serum electrolyte analysis suggests hypernatraemia. Which of the following conditions is most likely to be associated with hypernatraemia?**

- ○ A Syndrome of inappropriate antidiuretic hormone secretion (SIADH)
- ○ B Oedematous conditions
- ○ C Patients on diuretic therapy
- ○ D Patients on osmotic cathartics
- ○ E Cases of water intoxication

3.11 **While playing football a 25-year-old man is kicked on the thigh by a player from the opposite team. The skin is not broken. Within 48 hours he notices a 6 x 8 cm purple patch at the site of injury. Which of the following substances most likely has to accumulate at the site of injury to produce a yellow-brown colour 2 weeks after the injury?**

- A   Lipofuscin
- B   Bilirubin
- C   Haemosiderin
- D   Melanin
- E   Glycogen

3.12 **Which of the following statements about special total parenteral nutrition (TPN) solutions is contrary to the available scientific evidence?**

- A   For patients in cardiac failure the TPN solution must be more concentrated
- B   Patients in renal failure who cannot be dialysed should be given a TPN solution without amino acids
- C   Patients in hepatic encephalopathy should receive branched-chain amino acids
- D   Hepatic failure patients should receive major calories in the form of intravenous glucose infusions
- E   Patients with respiratory failure may benefit from the replacement of some glucose energy intake with fat

3.13 **For which of the following conditions is morphine the analgesic of choice?**

- A   Head injuries
- B   Acute myocardial infarction
- C   Chronic obstructive pulmonary disease (COPD)
- D   Addison's disease
- E   Liver disease

pathology

3.14 **A patient presents in A&E with chemical burns involving his hands. Which of the following statements correctly describes the management of chemical burns?**

○ A   Chemical burns are usually superficial burns

○ B   Chemical burns must not be washed with water

○ C   Chemical burns should be treated with neutralising agents because they completely remove the causative chemical agents

○ D   Chemical burns may be aggravated by the use of neutralising agents

○ E   Chemical burns never progress with time

3.15 **You are managing a patient with bladder rupture in A&E. Which of the following statements about bladder rupture is contrary to the existing knowledge on the subject?**

○ A   Bladder rupture occurs extraperitoneally as a result of perforations by adjacent bony fragments from the site of pelvic fracture

○ B   Bladder rupture, if extraperitoneal, may be treated with prolonged Foley catheter drainage

○ C   Bladder rupture is often a result of straddle injury

○ D   Bladder rupture is diagnosed by cystography

○ E   Bladder rupture in association with severe pelvic fractures and massive retroperitoneal bleeding is best managed conservatively

pathology

3.16 **Which of the following statements about diagnosis and management of pancreatic trauma is correct?**

○ A   Signs of peritonitis develop early after blunt pancreatic trauma

○ B   Diagnostic peritoneal lavage is the investigation of choice for pancreatic trauma

○ C   Hyperamylasaemia is an indicator of pancreatic trauma

○ D   Ductal transection in the body of the pancreas is an indication for Whipple's procedure

○ E   Pancreatic fistulae originating from the parenchyma exclusive of the main duct in the body or head never close spontaneously

3.17 **A 25-year-old man presents in A&E with clinical signs and symptoms suggestive of hepatic trauma. Which of the following features will prompt the consultant to opt for an immediate operation?**

○ A   Intrahepatic haematoma seen on computed tomography (CT) that is non-expanding

○ B   No evidence of active bleeding

○ C   A non-bleeding laceration of the liver seen on CT with associated splenic trauma

○ D   A laceration < 3 cm in parenchymal depth

○ E   A subcapsular haematoma involving 10–50% surface area

3.18 **After blunt abdominal trauma diagnostic peritoneal lavage is indicated:**

○ A   In a patient with an altered sensorium from a head injury

○ B   In a patient with a previous midline laparotomy scar

○ C   In a patient with significant haematoma of the abdominal wall related to pelvic fracture

○ D   In the latter stages of pregnancy

○ E   In a patient with morbid obesity

pathology

3.19 Which of the following changes is most likely to be seen after major trauma?

○   A   There is profound insulin hypersensitivity

○   B   Marked vasoconstriction occurs in vessels that perfuse injured areas during the hyperdynamic phase

○   C   Peripheral resistance increases

○   D   Control of wound circulation is different to other critical tissues

○   E   The liver is the origin of the nitrogen loss in the urine

3.20 Which of the following statements correctly describes the approach to a patient with trauma to the neck?

○   A   A radiograph of the neck is a particularly useful diagnostic tool for suspected laryngeal fracture or penetrating laryngeal injury

○   B   Zone I or thoracic inlet injuries must be investigated with panendoscopy and early arteriography

○   C   Zone II injuries are injuries to the upper neck

○   D   Zone III injuries must be immediately explored without any preliminary investigations

○   E   Zone III extends from the clavicular heads to the angles of the jaw

pathology

3.21 A 56-year-old man with past history of heavy alcohol consumption has been treated in the hospital for pancreatitis for the past 3 weeks. He is examined one morning on rounds and found to have a swollen right leg. It is tender to palpation posteriorly but is not warm. This condition is most likely to be the result of which of the following pathological processes?

○ A Septic embolisation
○ B Congestive heart failure
○ C Venous thrombosis
○ D Cellulitis
○ E Infarction

3.22 An 80-year-old woman was hospitalised after a fall from steps that resulted in fracture of the neck of the femur on the right side. After surgery to replace the broken hip she was bedridden and was unable to ambulate until about a month later, when she died suddenly. Which of the following conditions is most likely to be the immediate cause of her death?

○ A Carcinoma of the uterus
○ B TB
○ C Pneumococcal pneumonia
○ D Pulmonary embolism
○ E Congestive heart failure

pathology

3.23 **A 25-year-old man is involved in a motor vehicle accident that results in a compound fracture of the left femur, along with blunt abdominal trauma. In A&E he is noted to have cool, pallid skin. He has vital signs showing: temperature 36.7°C, pulse 103/min, respiratory rate 18/min and blood pressure (BP) 70/30 mmHg. He has decreased urine output. Which of the following laboratory findings on a blood sample from this patient is most likely to be present?**

- A Haematocrit of 42%
- B Glucose of 40 mg/dl
- C P_{AO_2} of 2.7 kPa (20 mmHg)
- D Troponin I of 4 ng/ml
- E Lactic acid of 4.8 mmol/l

3.24 **A 25-year-old man suffered a traumatic blow to his right forearm while playing football. He was referred to an orthopaedics outpatient clinic after he continued to have pain and tenderness 3 months later. A plain film radiograph revealed a 4-cm circumscribed mass in the soft tissue adjacent to the radius. The mass contained areas of brightness on the radiograph. The consultant reassured him that it was nothing sinister. Over the next year this process gradually resolved. Which of the following terms best describes this process?**

- A Dysplasia
- B Metaplasia
- C Hyperplasia
- D Hypertrophy
- E Neoplasia

3.25 A young patient is diagnosed with a neurofibroma. Which of the following statements best describes neurofibroma?

○ A   A neurofibroma arises from the connective tissue of the nerve sheath

○ B   A neurofibroma presents as a smooth, firm, 'painful subcutaneous nodule' which can be moved along the line of the nerve from which it arises

○ C   A neurofibroma can be easily removed from the nerve from which it arises

○ D   Plexiform neurofibromatosis is a rare condition characterised by multiple malignant neurofibromas

○ E   A neurofibroma along with pigmentation (café au lait) of the skin is a feature of Ollier's disease

3.26 Which of the following statements about spread of malignant tumours is correct?

○ A   Permeation means that cancer cells that invade a lymphatic vessel can break away and be carried by lymph circulation to a regional node

○ B   Malignant melanoma spreads by permeation alone

○ C   'Kiss cancer' of the labium majus is an example of spread of malignant tumours by implantation

○ D   Krukenberg's tumour is an example of haematogenous spread

○ E   Rodent ulcer spreads via the lymphatics

pathology

3.27 A 36-year-old woman presents with a trophic ulcer over the ball of the big toe of her left foot. Which of the following conditions is least likely to be diagnosed in this patient?

- ○ A   Chronic vasospasm
- ○ B   Syringomyelia
- ○ C   Diabetes
- ○ D   Spina bifida
- ○ E   TB

3.28 A 53-year-old woman with a history of full-thickness burn involving her right forearm presented in a surgical outpatient clinic with a Marjolin's ulcer. Which of the following statements best describes a Marjolin's ulcer?

- ○ A   It is a sarcoma that develops in a scar
- ○ B   It grows rapidly
- ○ C   It is painless
- ○ D   It is usually associated with secondary deposits in the regional lymph nodes
- ○ E   It is due to localized areas of fat necrosis.

3.29 A 22-year-old man who had previously undergone laparotomy for removal of a malignant growth involving the small bowel has now got a persistent sinus in his midline laparotomy scar. Which of the following conditions is least likely to be associated with persistence of a sinus?

○ A Presence of a foreign body or necrotic tissue
○ B Inefficient or non-dependent drainage
○ C Unrelieved obstruction of the lumen of a viscus
○ D Excess vitamin C intake
○ E Irradiation

3.30 A child is diagnosed with xeroderma pigmentosum. Which of the following statements best describes this disorder?

○ A Xeroderma pigmentosum is associated with increased incidence of bladder cancer
○ B Xeroderma pigmentosum is characterised by defective DNA repair
○ C Xeroderma pigmentosum leads to failure of antigen presentation by Langerhans' cells of the skin
○ D Xeroderma pigmentosum is a sex-linked disorder
○ E Xeroderma pigmentosum-associated tumours are caused by reverse transcriptase-mediated copying of the viral RNA genome

pathology

3.31 A 28-year-old man of south Asian origin has had a chronic cough with fever for 2 months. On physical examination his temperature is 37.9°C. A chest radiograph reveals a diffuse bilateral reticulonodular pattern. A transbronchial biopsy is performed. On microscopic examination of the biopsy there are focal areas of inflammation containing epithelioid macrophages, Langhans' giant cells and lymphocytes. These findings are most typical for which of the following immunological responses?

○　A　Type IV hypersensitivity
○　B　Type I hypersensitivity
○　C　Type II hypersensitivity
○　D　Graft-versus-host disease
○　E　Polyclonal B-cell activation

3.32 A 22-year-old man with previous history of corrective cardiac surgery in infancy is given intravenous penicillin to treat infective endocarditis. Within minutes of starting this therapy, he begins to have severe difficulty breathing with respiratory stridor and tachypnoea. He suddenly develops an erythematous skin rash over most of his body. His symptoms are most likely to be produced by release of which of the following chemical mediators?

○　A　Interleukin-1 (IL-1)
○　B　Histamine
○　C　Bradykinin
○　D　Complement C5a
○　E　Thromboxane

3.33 **After suturing of surgical wounds a substance, produced by macrophages, is found at the wound site which stimulates capillary proliferation during the first week. Which of the following substances is most likely to have this function?**

○ A Platelet-derived growth factor
○ B Phospholipase Cγ
○ C Fibroblast growth factor
○ D Fibronectin
○ E Epidermal growth factor

3.34 **After a laparotomy almost all of the tensile strength that can be obtained in wound healing in the skin will most probably be achieved within which of the following time periods?**

○ A One week
○ B One month
○ C Three months
○ D Six months
○ E One year

3.35 **A 20-year-old man had his thymus removed through a median sternotomy. Two months later there is a firm, 4 x 3 cm nodular mass with intact overlying epithelium in the region of the incision. On examination the scar is firm, but not tender, with no erythema. This mass is excised and micro-scopically shows fibroblasts with abundant collagen. Which of the following mechanisms has most probably produced this series of events?**

○ A Development of a fibrosarcoma
○ B Poor wound healing
○ C Keloid formation
○ D Foreign body response from suturing
○ E Staphylococcal wound infection

pathology

3.36 A 52-year-old woman was investigated for vague abdominal discomfort of 4 months' duration. Her clinical examination was negative for lymphadenopathy, abdominal masses or organomegaly. Bowel sounds were audible. A stool specimen tested for occult blood was negative. Abdominal CT showed a 20-cm retroperitoneal soft tissue mass obscuring the left psoas muscle. Which of the following neoplasms is this woman most likely to have?

○ A   Melanoma
○ B   Liposarcoma
○ C   Hamartoma
○ D   Adenocarcinoma
○ E   Lymphoma

3.37 A fine-needle aspiration (FNA) biopsy is performed of a 2-cm firm mass in the right breast of a 45-year-old woman. On microscopic examination a ductal carcinoma is seen. A poorer prognosis for the patient is most closely associated with which of the following findings?

○ A   Positive immunohistochemical staining for oestrogen receptors
○ B   A well-differentiated histological appearance
○ C   Intraductal growth pattern
○ D   Stage $T_1 N_0 M_0$
○ E   Aneuploidy by flow cytometry

3.38 A 45-year-old woman has had increasing cold intolerance, weight gain of 5 kg and sluggishness over the past 2 years. A physical examination reveals dry, coarse skin and alopecia of the scalp. Her thyroid is not palpably enlarged. Her serum thyroid-stimulating hormone (TSH) is 11.7 mU/l with thyroxine (T4) of 2.1 µg/dl. A year ago, anti-thyroglobulin and anti-microsomal autoantibodies were detected at high titre. Which of the following thyroid diseases is she most likely to have?

○ A   Hashimoto's thyroiditis
○ B   DeQuervain's disease
○ C   Papillary carcinoma
○ D   Medullary thyroid carcinoma
○ E   Graves' disease

3.39 An 82-year-old woman with no major medical problems is evaluated in A&E after a fall with a painful left hip and an inability to ambulate. Radiographs show not only a fracture of the left femoral head, but also a compressed fracture of the T10 vertebra. Which of the following conditions is she most likely to have?

○ A   Acute osteomyelitis
○ B   Osteogenesis imperfecta
○ C   Osteoporosis
○ D   Polyostotic fibrous dysplasia
○ E   Metastatic breast carcinoma

pathology

3.40 A 14-year-old girl complains of pain persisting in her right leg for 4 weeks. On physical examination her temperature is 37.9°C. A radiograph of the leg reveals a mass in the diaphyseal region of the left femur with overlying cortical erosion and soft tissue extension. A bone biopsy is performed and the lesion shows numerous small round blue cells on microscopic examination. Which of the following neoplasms is she most likely to have?

○ A Medulloblastoma
○ B Neuroblastoma
○ C Chondroblastoma
○ D Osteoblastoma
○ E Ewing's sarcoma

3.41 A 19-year-old boy who is a rugby player has noted pain in his right knee after each practice session for the past 2 months. On examination there is tenderness to palpation of his right knee, with reduced range of motion. A plain film of the right leg reveals a mass of the proximal tibial metaphysis that erodes the bone cortex, lifting up the periosteum where reactive new bone is apparent. The mass does not extend into the epiphyseal region. A bone biopsy is performed and microscopic examination shows atypical, elongated cells with hyperchromatic nuclei in an osteoid stroma. Which of the following neoplasms is he most likely to have?

○ A Metastatic seminoma
○ B Ewing's sarcoma
○ C Chondrosarcoma
○ D Osteosarcoma
○ E Multiple myeloma

pathology

3.42 A 47-year-old man who is a heavy alcohol drinker presents in A&E with massive haematemesis after a prolonged bout of vomiting. His vital signs are temperature 36.7°C, pulse 112/min, respiratory rate 23/min and BP 80/40 mmHg. His heart has a regular rate and rhythm with no murmurs, and his lungs are clear to auscultation. His abdominal examination is unremarkable. His stool is negative for occult blood. Which of the following is the most likely diagnosis?

○　A　Oesophageal pulsion diverticulum

○　B　Oesophageal squamous cell carcinoma

○　C　Oesophageal laceration (Mallory–Weiss syndrome)

○　D　Barrett's oesophagus

○　E　Hiatus hernia

3.43 A 50-year-old man with complaints of vague abdominal pain, unrelieved by over-the-counter antacid medications, and nausea for the past 3 years had an upper GI endoscopy after an unremarkable clinical examination. The endoscopy revealed antral mucosal erythema, but no ulcerations or masses. Microscopic examination of the biopsies showed a chronic non-specific gastritis. Which of the following conditions is most likely to be present in this man?

○　A　Zollinger–Ellison syndrome

○　B　*Helicobacter pylori* infection

○　C　Pernicious anaemia

○　D　Linitis plastica

○　E　Crohn's disease

pathology

3.44 A 27-year-old man has experienced low-grade fevers, night sweats and generalised malaise for the past 3 months. On physical examination he has non-tender cervical and supraclavicular lymphadenopathy. A cervical lymph node biopsy is performed. On microscopic examination at high magnification there are occasional Reed–Sternberg cells along with large and small lymphocytes and bands of fibrosis. Which of the following is the most likely diagnosis?

- ○ A Burkitt's lymphoma
- ○ B TB
- ○ C Mycosis fungoides
- ○ D Multiple myeloma
- ○ E Hodgkin's disease

3.45 A 32-year-old man with isolated enlargement of the left testis and a palpable left inguinal lymph node presents in a surgical outpatient clinic. He is advised to undergo scrotal ultrasonography. He also has a serum β-human chorionic gonadotrophin (βhCG) of 5 IU/l and α-fetoprotein (AFP) of 2 ng/ml. The left testis is removed on the next available operation list. Gross examination on sectioning reveals a firm, lobulated, light-tan mass without haemorrhage or necrosis. The consultant surgeon asks his senior house officer to refer this man for radiotherapy. Which of the following testicular tumours is he most likely to have?

- ○ A Seminoma
- ○ B Choriocarcinoma
- ○ C Embryonal carcinoma
- ○ D Yolk sac tumour
- ○ E Leydig's cell tumour

pathology

3.46 During physical examination for the purpose of life insurance, a 38-year-old man is found to have a left inguinal mass. The right testis is palpated in the scrotum and is of normal size, but a left testis cannot be palpated in the scrotum.
Ultrasonography shows that the inguinal mass is consistent with a cryptorchid testis. Which of the following approaches is most appropriate to deal with this patient's testicular abnormality?

○ A   Perform orchidopexy
○ B   Remove both testes
○ C   Commence testosterone therapy
○ D   Remove only the cryptorchid testis
○ E   Perform a chromosome analysis

3.47 A 78-year-old healthy man is noticed on a routine annual check-up to have a firm nodule palpable in the prostate on digital rectal examination. Microscopic examination of the biopsies of this nodule show small, crowded glands containing cells with prominent nucleoli in the nuclei. This man is most likely to have which of the following conditions?

○ A   Benign prostatic hyperplasia
○ B   Chronic prostatitis
○ C   Metastatic urothelial carcinoma
○ D   Infarction of the prostate
○ E   Adenocarcinoma of the prostate

3.48 After a bee sting adrenaline is injected to prevent:

○ A   Local immune complex formation
○ B   Systemic anaphylaxis
○ C   Interleukin release from macrophages
○ D   Binding of anti-receptor antibody
○ E   Complement activation

pathology

3.49 A 22-year-old woman has a solitary thyroid nodule. Which of the following statements about a solitary thyroid nodule is true?

○ A Hot nodules are much more likely to be neoplastic than cold ones

○ B Ultrasonography is a useful investigation for distinguishing cystic from solid lesions

○ C Excision biopsy has no role in the management of a solitary thyroid nodule

○ D The actual type of a neoplasm is always determined by FNA cytology (FNAC)

○ E Sudden increase in the size of a solitary nodule over a period of 24 hours is a definite sign of malignancy

3.50 Tamoxifen is a chemopreventive agent in breast cancer. Which of the following statements about tamoxifen is true?

○ A It causes breast epithelial cells to rest in G0 phase

○ B It is effective for women with hormone-receptor-negative breast cancer

○ C It has no effect on other body tissues and organs apart from the breast

○ D It is not effective in premenopausal patients

○ E It has side-effects similar to those of natural progesterone

3.51 **The histology report of a patient who had undergone surgery to remove a lump involving the right lobe of the thyroid gland came back as papillary carcinoma. Which of the following statements about this tumour is true?**

○   A   It is commonly seen only in old age

○   B   It classically presents with bone pain and tetany

○   C   It has a poor prognosis

○   D   It disseminates via the haematogenous route

○   E   It is treated by total thyroidectomy with preservation of the parathyroid glands

3.52 **A patient with fat malabsorption caused by biliary tract disease develops vitamin K deficiency. Which of the following clotting factors will not be carboxylated in this patient?**

○   A   Factor VII

○   B   Factor V

○   C   Factor XII

○   D   Factor XI

○   E   Factor VIII

3.53 **A patient with a defective neutrophil NADPH oxidase system will be unable to generate:**

○   A   Bactericidal permeability increasing protein

○   B   Reactive oxygen intermediates

○   C   Lysozyme

○   D   Major basic protein

○   E   Defensins

pathology

3.54 The critical step in the elaboration of the biological functions of complement is the activation of:

○　A　C1

○　B　C2

○　C　C3

○　D　C4

○　E　C5

3.55 The intrinsic clotting pathway is triggered by activation of Hageman factor (factor XII) on contact with negatively charged surfaces, such as collagen and basement membranes. Which other system is triggered by activation of factor XII?

○　A　Complement system

○　B　Renin–angiotensin system

○　C　Cyclo-oxygenase pathway

○　D　Kinin system

○　E　Lipoxygenase pathway

3.56 A 72-year-old woman is diagnosed with carcinoma of the gallbladder. Which of the following statements about this tumour is true?

○　A　Carcinoma of the gallbladder predominantly affects males

○　B　Gallstones are not associated with this tumour

○　C　At the time of diagnosis most tumours are limited to the gallbladder

○　D　Of the tumours, 95% are squamous cell carcinomas

○　E　The 5-year survival rate is 1% despite surgical intervention

3.57 **A 35-year-old man presented with a painless, slow-growing, mobile, discrete mass within the superficial lobe of the parotid gland. He underwent superficial parotidectomy. Histology of the mass showed epithelial elements dispersed within a mesenchyme-like background of loose myxoid tissue containing islands of cartilage and foci of bone. This patient is most likely to have:**

- A   Oncocytoma
- B   Warthin's tumour
- C   Pleomorphic adenoma
- D   Basal cell adenoma
- E   Canalicular adenoma

3.58 **Three days after a fracture of the right femur and tibia, a patient on the orthopaedic ward was noticed to develop sudden onset of tachypnoea, dyspnoea and tachycardia, accompanied by progressive delirium and a diffuse petechial rash in non-dependent areas. This clinical picture is suggestive of:**

- A   Pulmonary embolism
- B   Fat embolism
- C   Disseminated intravascular coagulation
- D   Air embolism
- E   Systemic thromboembolism

pathology

3.59 Mast cells have cytoplasmic membrane-bound granules that contain a variety of biologically active mediators. Which of the following is a mediator contained within mast-cell granules?

○ A   Chondroitin sulphate
○ B   Leukotriene C_4 (LTC$_4$)
○ C   Prostaglandin D_2
○ D   Platelet-activating factor
○ E   IL-1

3.60 Which of the following cytokines is an endogenous pyrogen?

○ A   Transforming growth factor-β
○ B   IL-2
○ C   Interferon-γ
○ D   IL-1
○ E   IL-6

3.61 Which of the following is an acute-phase protein?

○ A   IL-1
○ B   Tumour necrosis factor (TNF)
○ C   IL-6
○ D   IL-2
○ E   Fibrinogen

pathology

3.62 A 40-year-old woman with orthostatic hypotension is suspected of having primary hypoaldosteronism. Which of the following laboratory values will substantiate this diagnosis?

		Serum Na⁺	Serum K⁺	Serum HCO₃⁻	Urine Na⁺	Urine K⁺
○	A	Decreased	Increased	Decreased	Increased	Decreased
○	B	Decreased	Increased	Increased	Increased	Decreased
○	C	Decreased	Decreased	Decreased	Increased	Increased
○	D	Increased	Decreased	Increased	Decreased	Increased
○	E	Increased	Increased	Increased	Decreased	Decreased

3.63 A 62-year-old man is brought to A&E after a sudden myocardial infarction. On arrival he is in pulmonary oedema with an audible third heart sound and distended jugular veins. His ECG shows prominent Q waves in the lateral chest leads. Which of the following haemodynamic parameters will be consistent with this patient's condition?

		Preload	Cardiac output	PAWP	CVP	Vascular resistance	Mixed venous O₂
○	A	Decreased	Decreased	Increased	Decreased	Decreased	Decreased
○	B	Increased	Decreased	Increased	Increased	Increased	Decreased
○	C	Increased	Decreased	Decreased	Increased	Increased	Decreased
○	D	Increased	Increased	Decreased	Decreased	Decreased	Increased
○	E	Decreased	Increased	Decreased	Decreased	Decreased	Increased

CVP, central venous pressure; PAWP, pulmonary artery wedge pressure.

pathology

3.64 **A severely ill patient in septic shock after a perforated duodenal ulcer develops acute renal failure with azotaemia and oliguria. The urine osmolality approaches that of the glomerular ultrafiltrate. A renal biopsy would be most likely to show which of the following?**

○ A Acute pyelonephritis

○ B Renal cell carcinoma

○ C Acute tubular necrosis

○ D Crescentic glomerulonephritis

○ E Chronic glomerulonephritis

3.65 **A 35-year-old woman who is a secretary develops a pea-sized, translucent nodule on the wrist, which when excised shows cystic degeneration without a true cell lining. Which of the following is the most probable diagnosis?**

○ A Villonodular synovitis

○ B Synovial cyst

○ C Rheumatoid nodule

○ D Ganglion cyst

○ E Gout

3.66 **A 28-year-old man with a history of significant weight loss and drenching night sweats presents to his general practitioner with a lump in the left side of his neck. He is referred for biopsy of the mass, which reveals Reed–Sternberg cells. Further evaluation after the biopsy report shows nodal involvement limited to the neck and axilla. What stage of disease has he got?**

- ○ A IA
- ○ B IB
- ○ C IIA
- ○ D IIB
- ○ E IIIB

3.67 **A 24-year-old woman presents in a surgical outpatient clinic with paraesthesia of the right shoulder and arm. On palpation a hard bony structure is noticed above the clavicle on the affected side. Which of the following conditions best accounts for her symptoms?**

- ○ A Osteoporosis
- ○ B Pancoast's tumour
- ○ C Shoulder dislocation
- ○ D Horner's syndrome
- ○ E Thoracic outlet obstruction

pathology

3.68 **A 15-year-old girl complains of fatigue and palpitations. Clinical examination shows pale mucous membranes and a systolic murmur. A peripheral blood smear shows hypochromic/microcytic red blood cells. Which of the following is the most likely diagnosis?**

○ A Iron deficiency

○ B Folate deficiency

○ C Sickle cell anaemia

○ D Vitamin B_{12} deficiency

○ E Hereditary spherocytosis

3.69 **After a total hip replacement a 72-year-old woman develops wound infection with methicillin-resistant *Staphylococcus aureus* (MRSA). Which of the following antibiotics will be effective against this bacterium?**

○ A Ampicillin

○ B Gentamicin

○ C Cefotaxime

○ D Cefazolin

○ E Vancomycin

3.70 **A patient treated for a life-threatening Gram-negative sepsis with an intravenous antibiotic complained of disturbed hearing and loss of balance. Which of the following antibiotics is responsible for this side-effect?**

○ A Amoxicillin

○ B Cefuroxime

○ C Cefotaxime

○ D Gentamicin

○ E Ciprofloxacin

pathology

3.71 **A patient admitted for elective cholecystectomy is detected as being infected with hepatitis B on preoperative screening. Which of the following serological markers signifies active viral replication in this patient?**

○ A HBsAg

○ B HBeAg

○ C IgM anti-HBc

○ D IgG anti-HBc

○ E IgG anti-HBs

3.72 **A variety of diseases has been found to be associated with certain HLA alleles. Which of the following disorders is associated with HLA-B27?**

○ A Chronic active hepatitis

○ B Postgonococcal arthritis

○ C Rheumatoid arthritis

○ D Primary Sjögren's syndrome

○ E Type 2 diabetes

3.73 **A 65-year-old man, who is a smoker and has intermittent haematuria and costovertebral pain, presents in A&E with haemoptysis. On clinical examination, there is a palpable mass in the left flank and his laboratory investigations show polycythaemia, hypercalcaemia and eosinophilia. Which of the following is the most likely diagnosis in this man?**

○ A Oncocytoma of the left kidney

○ B Angiomyolipoma of the left kidney

○ C Renal cell carcinoma of the left kidney

○ D Renal hamartoma of the left kidney

○ E Wilms' tumour of the left kidney

pathology

3.74 **The measurement of the serum TSH concentration using sensitive TSH assays provides the most useful single screening test for hyperthyroidism. Which of the following combinations of TSH and T_4 levels suggest hyperthyroidism?**

○ A Low TSH, low T_4
○ B High TSH, normal T_4
○ C Normal TSH, low T_4
○ D Low TSH, high T_4
○ E High TSH, high T_4

3.75 **Which of the following is a tumour-suppressor gene?**

○ A *S/S*
○ B *INT–2*
○ C *HST–1*
○ D *HGF*
○ E *P53*

3.76 **Chloride-responsive metabolic alkalosis (urine chloride < 20 mmol/l) is seen in:**

○ A Loss of gastric secretions
○ B Adrenal adenoma
○ C Liddle's syndrome
○ D Congenital adrenal hyperplasia
○ E Bartter's syndrome

pathology

3.77 **The histopathology report of a patient with papillary carcinoma of urinary bladder indicates muscularis propria invasion with no nodes or distant spread. How would you stage this tumour?**

○   A   Stage I
○   B   Stage II
○   C   Stage III
○   D   Stage IV
○   E   Stage 0a

3.78 **A 29-year-old woman presents with weight loss, abdominal pain and bloody diarrhoea. Sigmoidoscopy/colonoscopy reveals mucosal erythema and ulceration extending in a continuous fashion proximally from the rectum. Which of the following pathological findings would also be characteristic of this patient's condition?**

○   A   Bowel wall thickening
○   B   Fistulae
○   C   Pseudopolyps
○   D   Transmural lesions
○   E   Cobblestone appearance of the mucosa

3.79 **The hypocalcaemia in acute pancreatitis reflects:**

○   A   Gangrenous necrosis
○   B   Caseous necrosis
○   C   Coagulative necrosis
○   D   Enzymatic fat necrosis
○   E   Liquefactive necrosis

pathology

3.80 From a clinical standpoint, tumours of the testis are segregated into two broad categories: seminomas and non-seminomatous germ-cell tumours (NSGCTs). Which of the following statements about NSGCTs is true?

○ A These tumours tend to remain localised to the testis for a long time

○ B These tumours do not metastasise

○ C These tumours are radiosensitive

○ D These tumours are less aggressive

○ E These tumours have a poorer prognosis

3.81 A 45-year-old man who smokes 30 cigarettes a day is diagnosed with a non-small-cell lung cancer. On CT he has a 4-cm tumour involving the left upper lobe bronchus, which is > 2 cm from the carina. What tumour stage has this man got, according to the TNM staging system?

○ A T_{IS}

○ B T_1

○ C T_2

○ D T_3

○ E T_4

3.82 A 35-year-old man who has been a heavy smoker for the last 18 years complains of severe pain in both legs even at rest and has chronic ulceration of his toes. Which of the following conditions is he most likely to have?

○ A Wegener's granulomatosis

○ B Buerger's disease

○ C Kawasaki's disease

○ D Polyarteritis nodosa

○ E Takayasu's arteritis

3.83 Hamartomatous polyps in the colon are a feature of:

○ A   Peutz–Jeghers syndrome

○ B   Familial adenomatous polyposis syndrome

○ C   Gardner's syndrome

○ D   Turcot's syndrome

○ E   Lynch's syndrome

3.84 Which of the following is a seronegative spondyloarthropathy?

○ A   Osteoarthritis

○ B   Rheumatoid arthritis

○ C   Tuberculous arthritis

○ D   Lyme arthritis

○ E   Psoriatic arthritis

3.85 Immediate hypersensitivity reactions involve primary as well as secondary mediators. Which of the following substances is a secondary mediator of inflammation?

○ A   Histamine

○ B   Prostaglandin D_2

○ C   Chondroitin sulphate

○ D   Chymase

○ E   Tryptase

pathology

3.86 **The appendicectomy specimen from a 64-year-old woman was sent for histology because there was a suspicion that the bulbous swelling in the tip may be a carcinoid tumour. The histology report confirmed the diagnosis. Which of the following statements about carcinoid tumours of the appendix is correct?**

○ A The appendix is the most common site of gut carcinoid tumours

○ B All appendiceal carcinoids are symptomatic

○ C Of appendiceal carcinoids 90% metastasise

○ D All appendiceal carcinoids are associated with carcinoid syndrome

○ E The overall 5-year survival rate for carcinoid tumours is less than 20%

3.87 **Primary gastrointestinal lymphomas usually arise as sporadic neoplasms but also occur more frequently in certain patient populations. Which of the following patient populations is least likely to have primary gastrointestinal lymphomas?**

○ A Chronic gastritis caused by *Helicobacter pylori*

○ B Chronic sprue-like syndromes

○ C Native inhabitants of sub-Saharan Africa

○ D Congenital immunodeficiency states

○ E Infection with human immunodeficiency virus (HIV)

pathology

3.88 **A 35-year-old woman with progressive weakness and easy fatiguability for the last 6 months is seen in A&E complaining of anorexia, nausea, vomiting, weight loss and diarrhoea of 1 month's duration. On examination she is noticed to have hypotension and hyperpigmentation of the skin. Laboratory tests show hyperkalaemia, hyponatraemia and hypoglycaemia. What is the most likely diagnosis in this case?**

○ A Hypothyroidism
○ B Addison's disease
○ C SIADH
○ D Diabetes insipidus
○ E Primary hyperaldosteronism

3.89 **Which of the following drugs exerts a protective effect against colon cancer?**

○ A Methotrexate
○ B Cyclophosphamide
○ C Tamoxifen
○ D Etoposide
○ E Aspirin

3.90 **Povidone–iodine surgical scrub is used as an antiseptic skin cleanser for preoperative scrubbing and washing by surgeons and theatre staff and preoperative preparation of patients' skin. Which of the following statements about povidone–iodine is true?**

○ A It is a quaternary ammonium compound
○ B It acts by disrupting the bacterial cell wall
○ C It is bacteriostatic
○ D It is active against spore-forming organisms
○ E It acts by denaturing proteins

pathology

3.91 **A 48-year-old man notices a lump in the subcutaneous tissue in his left thigh. The lesion is removed. He is very relieved to learn that it is benign. Which of the following characteristics of this lesion would tend to point towards a benign neoplasm rather than a malignant one?**

○ A Infiltration of the surrounding tissues

○ B Well-defined encapsulation

○ C Prominent mitotic figures

○ D Anaplasia

○ E Metastasis

3.92 **A few weeks after an episode of group A streptococcal pharyngitis, a 12-year-old boy develops acute rheumatic fever. During the acute phase of the rheumatic fever, the characteristic inflammatory lesions found in his heart are known as:**

○ A Ferruginous bodies

○ B Foamy macrophages

○ C Langhans' giant cells

○ D Pyogenic granuloma

○ E Aschoff's bodies

3.93 **Which of the following interleukins is involved in B-cell, T-cell and natural killer (NK) cell survival, development and homeostasis?**

○ A IL-1

○ B IL-2

○ C IL-3

○ D IL-7

○ E IL-8

pathology

3.94 **The full blood count of a 35-year-old woman with respiratory complaints shows neutrophilic leukocytosis. Which of the following is associated with neutrophilic leukocytosis?**

- ○ A Hay fever
- ○ B Asthma
- ○ C Streptococcal pneumonia
- ○ D Ascaris infestation
- ○ E Loeffler's syndrome

3.95 **A sputum sample collected from a 65-year-old man with lobar pneumonia was subjected to a Gram-staining technique. Gram-positive, capsulated, flame-shaped diplococci were seen when the stained smear was examined under the microscope. Sputum culture on blood agar revealed dome-shaped, centrally umbilicated colonies with evidence of a haemolysis. The organism causing the infection is likely to be:**

- ○ A *Streptococcus pneumoniae*
- ○ B *Staphylococcus aureus*
- ○ C *Mycoplasma pneumoniae*
- ○ D *Klebsiella pneumoniae*
- ○ E *Corynebacterium diphtheriae*

pathology

3.96 A 60-year-old man with obstructive jaundice is diagnosed with infiltrating ductal adenocarcinoma of the pancreas. Which of the following statements about this tumour is true?

○ A About 60% of cancers of the pancreas arise in the body of the gland

○ B The *APC* gene is the most frequently altered oncogene in pancreatic cancer

○ C Carcinomas of the pancreas present very early with obstructive jaundice

○ D More than 50% of pancreatic cancers overall are resectable at the time of diagnosis

○ E The 5-year survival rate is less than 5%

3.97 A 65-year-old man underwent right hemicolectomy for a carcinoma involving the ascending colon. Preoperative assessment showed no evidence of metastatic spread. The resected specimen along with lymph nodes in the mesentery was sent for histopathology reporting. The report received a week later read: the specimen of large bowel on gross examination had a polypoid, exophytic mass that extends along one wall of the capacious caecum and ascending colon for about 6 cm. On microscopy the adenocarcinoma is extending into the muscularis propria but not penetrating through it. Five of the seven nodes in mesentery have metastatic deposits. Using the TNM staging system what would you stage this tumour as?

○ A Stage IIA

○ B Stage IIB

○ C Stage IIIA

○ D Stage IIIB

○ E Stage IIIC

pathology

3.98 **Monoclonal antibodies are used to detect serum antigens associated with specific malignancies. These tumour markers are most useful for monitoring response to therapy and detecting early relapse. Which of the following tumour markers is used to follow response to therapy in patients with metastatic breast cancer?**

○ A CEA
○ B CA-27.29
○ C CA-19-9
○ D CA-125
○ E AFP

3.99 **Immediately after elective right hemicolectomy the catabolic phase is characterised by:**

○ A Increased metabolic demands
○ B Mobilisation of glucose to serve as a substrate for gluconeogenesis
○ C Decreased urinary nitrogen excretion
○ D Decreased fatty acid oxidation
○ E Increased response to insulin

3.100 **Synovial fluid analysis is commonly performed to determine the cause of acute arthritis. Which of the following synovial fluid analysis findings is correctly associated with the causative lesion?**

○ A High viscosity in tuberculous arthritis
○ B Turbid appearance in rheumatoid arthritis
○ C Thin, needle-shaped, negatively birefringent crystals in pseudogout
○ D 200–2000 white blood cells/mm^3 in osteoarthritis
○ E > 75% polymorphonuclear leukocytes in psoriatic arthritis

pathology

ANSWERS

SECTION 1:
ANATOMY – ANSWERS

1.1

Answer: B

The axillary artery, the continuation of the subclavian, commences at the outer border of the first rib and ends at the lower border of the tendon of teres major, where it takes the name of brachial. At its origin the artery is very deeply situated, but near its termination it is superficial, being covered only by skin and fascia. To facilitate the description of the vessel it is divided into three portions: the first lies above, the second behind and the third below pectoralis minor. The branches of the axillary artery are: from the first part, the superior thoracic artery; from the second part, the thoracoacromial artery and lateral thoracic artery; and from the third part, the subscapular artery, posterior humeral circumflex artery and anterior humeral circumflex artery. The anterior and posterior circumflex humeral branches supply the humerus.

1.2

Answer: E

Flexion at the elbow is produced by biceps brachii and brachialis; both of these muscles are innervated by the musculocutaneous nerve, so it is evident that the musculocutaneous nerve has been damaged. Beyond innervating the muscles that flex the forearm, the musculocutaneous nerve gives off the lateral antebrachial cutaneous nerve that provides sensory innervation to the anterolateral surface of the forearm. This means that the other symptom that would be present is a loss of cutaneous sensation on the anterolateral surface of the forearm. The biceps brachii and coracobrachialis muscles flex the arm, so there should be weakening of flexion at the shoulder, although function of pectoralis major, a powerful arm flexor, must still be intact.

1.3

Answer: A

The lower subscapular nerve (C5, C6) supplies the lower part of subscapularis and ends in teres major; the latter is sometimes supplied by a separate branch. Teres minor and deltoid are supplied by the axillary nerve. The suprascapular nerve innervates the supraspinatus and infraspinatus muscles.

1.4

Answer: C

The femoral sheath is divided by two vertical partitions that stretch between its anterior and posterior walls. The lateral compartment contains the femoral artery, and the intermediate compartment contains the femoral vein, whereas the medial and smallest compartment is named the femoral canal, and contains some lymphatic vessels and a lymph gland embedded in a small amount of areolar tissue. The femoral canal is conical and measures about 1.25 cm in length.

1.5

Answer: E

The superficial peroneal nerve provides cutaneous innervation to the lower anterior third of the leg and the dorsum of the foot. It reaches the dorsum of the foot by crossing over the anterior midline of the ankle region. Both the area of injury and the subsequent symptoms should point to damage of the superficial peroneal nerve. The femoral nerve is mostly important as a motor nerve – it innervates quadriceps femoris, sartorius and pectineus. Its anterior femoral cutaneous branches provide sensory innervation to the medial and anterior thigh. Another branch of the femoral nerve, the saphenous nerve, provides sensory innervation to the medial side of the leg and foot. The lateral sural cutaneous nerve is a branch of the common peroneal nerve providing sensory innervation to the skin of the lateral side of the leg. The sural nerve, which runs down the posterior leg with the lesser saphenous vein, provides sensory innervation to the posterior surface of the lower leg and the lateral side of the foot.

1.6

Answer: E

Peroneal neuropathies are classically associated with external compression at the level of the fibular head. The most common aetiology is habitual leg crossing (which compresses this area). Prolonged positioning with pressure at this area (eg sitting on an airplane or positioning during surgery) are other causes. Short casts or braces around this area can be factors in external compression. Other causes include operative trauma (knee surgery), fibular fracture, blunt or open trauma, and intrinsic masses (eg ganglionic cysts, schwannoma). Lack or loss of the fat pad over the fibular head as a result of sudden weight loss and/or a thin body habitus predisposes the nerve to external compression at this site.

1.7

Answer: C

The thoracic duct conveys the greater part of the lymph and chyle into the blood. It is the common trunk of all the lymphatic vessels of the body, except those on the right side of the head, neck and thorax, and right upper extremity, the right lung, right side of the heart and convex surface of the liver. In the adult it varies in length from 38 to 45 cm and extends from the second lumbar vertebra to the root of the neck. It begins in the abdomen by a triangular dilatation, the cisterna chyli, which is situated on the front of the body of the second lumbar vertebra, to the right side of and behind the aorta, and by the side of the right crus of the diaphragm. It enters the thorax through the aortic hiatus of the diaphragm, and ascends through the posterior mediastinal cavity between the aorta and the azygos vein. It ends by opening into the angle of junction of the left subclavian vein with the left internal jugular vein. The thoracic duct has several valves; at its termination it is provided with a pair, the free borders of which are turned towards the vein, so as to prevent the passage of venous blood into the duct.

1.8

Answer: B

The anal canal below the pectinate line is supplied by the inferior rectal nerve (S2, S3, S4) and is responsible for the transmission of pain sensation. Anal fissure is caused by the rupture of one of the anal valves, usually by the passage of dry hard stool in someone who is constipated. Each valve is lined by mucous membrane above and skin below. As a result of skin involvement, the condition is extremely painful and associated with marked spasm of the anal sphincters.

1.9

Answer: E

The inguinal canal is an oblique canal about 4 cm long, slanting downwards and medially, and in parallel with and a little above the inguinal ligament; it extends from the abdominal inguinal ring to the subcutaneous inguinal ring. It is bounded by the integument and superficial fascia in front, by the aponeurosis of the external oblique throughout its whole length and by the internal oblique in its lateral third. It is bounded by: behind, the reflected inguinal ligament, the inguinal aponeurotic falx, the transversalis fascia, the extraperitoneal connective tissue and the peritoneum; above, the arched fibres of internal oblique and transversus abdominis; below, the union of the transversalis fascia with the inguinal ligament; and at its medial end, the lacunar ligament. The inguinal canal contains the spermatic cord and the ilioinguinal nerve in the male, and the round ligament of the uterus and the ilioinguinal nerve in the female.

1.10

Answer: C

The right bronchus receives blood from a single right bronchial artery. This artery may branch from one of the left bronchial arteries or from the right third posterior intercostal artery, the first intercostal artery that arises from the descending aorta. Damage of this artery might stop the blood supply to the main bronchus. The intercostal arteries to the first and second intercostal spaces are derived from the highest intercostal artery, so the blood supply to either of these spaces would not be disrupted. The left bronchus is supplied by two left bronchial arteries that branch directly from the descending aorta. The fibrous pericardium is a fibrous sac containing the pericardial cavity and the heart. Its blood supply is not a major concern, and is via branches from the internal mammary and musculophrenic arteries as well as from the descending thoracic aorta.

1.11

Answer: D

The diaphragm is pierced by a series of apertures to permit the passage of structures between the thorax and abdomen. Three large openings include the aortic, oesophageal and vena caval openings. The aortic hiatus is the lowest and most posterior of the large apertures; it lies at the level of the twelfth thoracic vertebra. Strictly speaking, it is not an aperture in the diaphragm but an osseo-aponeurotic opening between it and the vertebral column, and it is therefore behind the diaphragm. The aorta, azygos vein and thoracic duct pass through it; occasionally the azygos vein is transmitted via the right crus. The oesophageal hiatus is situated in the muscular part of the diaphragm at the level of the tenth thoracic vertebra; it is elliptical in shape. It is placed above, in front of and a little to the left of the aortic hiatus, and transmits the oesophagus, the vagus nerves and some small oesophageal arteries. The vena caval foramen is the highest of the three, and is situated at about the level of the fibrocartilage between the eighth and ninth thoracic vertebrae. It is quadrilateral in form, and is placed at the junction of the right and middle leaflets of the central tendon, so that its margins are tendinous. It transmits the inferior vena cava (IVC), the wall of which is adherent to the margins of the opening, and some branches of the right phrenic nerve.

1.12

Answer: B

The dorsal lingual artery runs on the superficial surface of the tongue – it is a branch of the lingual artery that delivers blood to the posterior superficial tongue. This artery must, therefore, be the source of the haemorrhage. The deep lingual and sublingual arteries are two terminal branches of the lingual artery. These branches run in the floor of the mouth (sublingual) and the deep surface of the tongue (deep lingual). The facial artery is a branch of the external carotid artery that courses across the face. The tonsillar artery is a branch of the facial artery that supplies blood to the palatine tonsil.

1.13

Answer: D

The left coronary artery, larger than the right, arises from the left anterior aortic sinus and divides into an anterior descending and a circumflex branch. The anterior descending branch passes at first behind the pulmonary artery, then coming forwards between that vessel and the left auricle to reach the anterior longitudinal sulcus, along which it descends to the apex of the heart; it gives branches to both ventricles. The circumflex branch follows the left part of the coronary sulcus, running first to the left and then to the right, reaching almost as far as the posterior longitudinal sulcus; it gives branches to the left atrium and ventricle. The left coronary artery supplies only a part of the left branch of the atrioventricular (AV) bundle (of His).

1.14

Answer: C

The abdominal portion of the oesophagus lies in the oesophageal groove on the posterior surface of the left lobe of the liver. It measures about 1.25 cm in length, and only its front and left aspects are covered by peritoneum. The arterial supply is mainly from the left gastric branch of the coeliac artery. The nerves are derived from the vagi and the sympathetic trunks; they form a plexus, in which there are groups of ganglion cells, between the two layers of the muscular coats, and also a second plexus in the submucous tissue.

anatomy

1.15

Answer: B

The taeniae coli are three bands of longitudinal muscle on the surface of the large intestine. Remember that the large intestine does not have a continuous layer of longitudinal muscle; instead, it has taeniae coli. The base of the appendix is fairly constant and is located at the posteromedial wall of the caecum about 2.5 cm below the ileocaecal valve. This is also where the taeniae converge. The base is at a constant location, whereas the position of the tip of the appendix varies. In 65% of patients, the tip is located in a retrocaecal position, in 30% it is located at the brim or in the true pelvis and in 5% it is extraperitoneal, situated behind the caecum, ascending colon or distal ileum. The location of the tip of the appendix determines early signs and symptoms in acute appendicitis. The appendix is below the ileocaecal valve, not above it. It is not near the right colic artery, which supplies the ascending colon. The appendix would not be found by removing a layer of the mesentery of the jejunoileum; in fact, the appendix has its own mesentery – the mesoappendix. Finally, the appendix is not on the pelvic brim.

1.16

Answer: D

The facial nerve consists of a motor and sensory part, the latter being frequently described under the name nervus intermedius. The two parts emerge at the lower border of the pons in the recess between the olive and the inferior peduncle. The motor part supplies somatic motor fibres to the muscles of the face, scalp and auricle, buccinator and platysma, stapedius, stylohyoid and the posterior belly of the digastric; it also contains some sympathetic motor fibres that constitute the vasodilator nerves of the submaxillary and sublingual glands; these are conveyed through the chorda tympani nerve. They are preganglionic fibres of the sympathetic system and terminate in the submaxillary ganglion and small ganglia in the hilus of the submaxillary gland. From these ganglia postganglionic fibres are conveyed to these glands. The sensory part contains the fibres of taste for the anterior two-thirds of the tongue and a few somatic sensory fibres from the middle-ear region. A few splanchnic sensory fibres are also present.

1.17

Answer: A

The descending portion (second part) of the duodenum is in relation, in front from above downwards, with the duodenal impression on the right lobe of the liver, the transverse colon and the small intestine; behind, it has a variable relation with the front of the right kidney in the neighbourhood of the hilum, and is connected to it by loose areolar tissue. The renal vessels, the IVC and the psoas muscle below are also behind it. At its medial side is the head of the pancreas and the common bile duct; to its lateral side is the right colic flexure.

1.18

Answer: D

The cystic artery, usually a branch of the right hepatic, passes downwards and forwards along the neck of the gallbladder, and divides into two branches, one of which ramifies on the free surface and the other on the attached surface of the gallbladder.

1.19

Answer: A

The femoral triangle is a depression seen immediately below the fold of the groin. Its apex is directed downwards; the sides are formed laterally by the medial margin of the sartorius, medially by the medial margin of adductor longus and above by the inguinal ligament. The floor of the space is formed from its lateral-to-medial side by iliacus, psoas major, pectineus, in some cases a small part of adductor brevis and adductor longus. It is divided into two almost equal parts by the femoral vessels, which extend from near the middle of its base to its apex: in this situation the artery gives off its superficial and profunda branches, the vein receiving the deep femoral and great saphenous tributaries. On the lateral side of the femoral artery is the femoral nerve, dividing into its branches. In addition to the vessels and nerves, this space contains some fat and lymphatics.

1.20

Answer: E

The adductor canal is an aponeurotic tunnel in the middle third of the thigh, extending from the apex of the femoral triangle to the opening in the adductor magnus. It is bounded, in front and laterally, by vastus medialis and, behind, by adductor longus and adductor magnus. It is covered in by a strong aponeurosis that extends from vastus medialis, across the femoral vessels to adductor longus and adductor magnus. Sartorius lies on the aponeurosis. The canal contains the femoral artery and vein, the saphenous nerve and the nerve to vastus medialis.

1.21

Answer: C

The lingual nerve is one of the two terminal branches of the posterior division of the mandibular nerve. It is sensory to the anterior two-thirds of the tongue and floor of the mouth. However, the fibres of the chorda tympani (branch of facial nerve), which is secretomotor to the submandibular and sublingual salivary glands and gustatory to the anterior two-thirds of the tongue, are also distributed through the lingual nerve. Lingual nerve injury, causing numbness, dysaesthesia, paraesthesia, and dysgeusia that involves the anterior two-thirds of the tongue, may complicate invasive dental and surgical procedures.

1.22

Answer: B

The superior gluteal artery, the largest branch of the internal iliac artery, appears to be a continuation of the posterior division of that vessel. It is a short artery that runs backwards between the lumbosacral trunk and the first sacral nerve; passing out of the pelvis above the upper border of the piriformis, it immediately divides into superficial and deep branches. Within the pelvis it gives off a few branches to iliacus, piriformis and obturator internus and, just before leaving that cavity, a nutrient artery that enters the ilium.

1.23

Answer: C

The anatomical snuffbox is a triangular depression on the lateral side of the wrist. It is seen best when the thumb is extended. It is bounded anteriorly by the tendons of abductor pollicis longus and extensor pollicis brevis, and posteriorly by the tendon of extensor pollicis longus. It is limited above by the styloid process of the radius. The floor of the snuffbox is formed by the scaphoid and trapezium, and it is crossed by the radial artery.

1.24

Answer: A

The musculocutaneous nerve arises from the lateral cord of the brachial plexus, opposite the lower border of pectoralis minor, its fibres being derived from the fifth, sixth and seventh cervical nerves. In its course through the arm, it supplies coracobrachialis, biceps brachii and the greater part of brachialis. Through the lateral cutaneous nerve of the forearm it supplies the skin of the lateral side of the forearm from the elbow to the wrist. Supinator is supplied by the posterior interosseus nerve.

1.25

Answer: B

The trochlear nerve (cranial nerve or CN IV) innervates the superior oblique muscle, so, to test this muscle, the eye needs to turn inwards (towards the nose) and downwards. The abducens nerve (CN VI) innervates the lateral rectus muscle. The oculomotor nerve (CN III) innervates the superior rectus, inferior rectus, medial rectus and inferior oblique muscles.

To understand this question, you need to understand how the motions of the eye are tested. As the actions of the extraocular muscles are complex, it is necessary to turn the eye to a position where a single action of each muscle predominates when evaluating the individual muscles. To test the superior and inferior recti, a patient needs to turn the eye outwards approximately 25°. At this

anatomy

position, the superior rectus will simply act to raise the eye and the inferior rectus to lower the eye. To test the superior and inferior obliques, a patient needs to turn the eye inwards about 50°. When the eye is in this position, the superior oblique muscle will act to lower the eye and the inferior oblique to raise the eye.

1.26

Answer: E

The internal branch of the superior laryngeal is a sensory nerve that pierces the thyrohyoid membrane along with the superior laryngeal artery. It supplies sensory fibres to the mucous membrane of the larynx, superior to the vocal folds. As this area has lost sensation, it appears that the internal branch of the superior laryngeal nerve must have been injured. The external branch of the superior laryngeal nerve is a motor nerve that innervates the cricothyroid muscle – it does not provide any sensory innervation to the larynx. The recurrent laryngeal nerve ascends from the thorax and provides motor innervation to the upper oesophagus, lower pharynx and all the laryngeal muscles except the cricothyroid muscle. The hypoglossal nerve supplies motor innervation to the muscles of the tongue. The lingual nerve is a sensory nerve for the anterior two-thirds of the tongue. These nerves are not important for innervating the larynx.

1.27

Answer: C

Damage to the recurrent laryngeal nerve is one possible cause of hoarseness. The recurrent laryngeal nerve changes its name to the inferior laryngeal nerve at the level of the inferior border of the cricoid cartilage. The inferior laryngeal nerve goes on to innervate all the intrinsic muscles of the larynx except cricothyroideus. So, if this nerve innervating all the muscles of the larynx were damaged, a patient would have a hoarse voice. The external and internal branches of the superior laryngeal nerve innervate cricothyroid, the inferior pharyngeal constrictor, and provide secretomotor fibres to mucosal glands of the larynx above the vocal folds. The pharyngeal branch of the glossopharyngeal nerve provides sensory innervation to the pharynx.

1.28

Answer: D

The auriculotemporal nerve is a branch of the mandibular division of the trigeminal nerve (V3). It has two important functions: first, it carries postganglionic parasympathetic fibres to the parotid gland. These fibres come from the otic ganglia, where they are synapsed with the presynaptic fibres from the glossopharyngeal nerve (CN IX). Second, the auriculotemporal nerve provides sensory innervation to the skin of the anterosuperior ear, part of the external auditory meatus and the temporomandibular joint. So, the listed symptoms match with an injury to the auriculotemporal nerve.

Chorda tympani is a branch of the facial nerve that provides secretomotor innervation to the submandibular and sublingual glands. It carries preganglionic parasympathetic axons to the submandibular ganglion. In the infratemporal fossa, chorda tympani joins the lingual nerve; it continues with the lingual nerve to the tongue where it supplies taste to the anterior two-thirds of the tongue. The posterior deep temporal nerve is a branch of the mandibular division of the trigeminal nerve, which supplies motor innervation to temporalis. The facial nerve (CN VII) innervates all the muscles of facial expression, and, through chorda tympani, provides secretomotor innervation to the submandibular and sublingual glands as well as taste sensation to the anterior two-thirds of the tongue. Finally, the great auricular nerve comes from the cervical plexus; it provides sensory innervation to the skin of the ear and the skin below the ear.

1.29

Answer: E

The sigmoid colon is the most likely intestinal segment to be involved in a left-sided indirect inguinal hernia, mainly because of its location but also because it has a mesentery. Although the descending colon is on the left side of the abdomen as well, it is slightly superior to be herniating through the deep inguinal ring. The ascending colon and caecum are on the right side of the abdomen, so they would not be involved in a left-sided hernia. Finally, the rectum is a structure in the pelvis; it is too inferior to enter the deep inguinal ring and cause an indirect inguinal hernia. Moreover, all of these structures lack a mesentery and hence are not mobile enough to herniate.

1.30

Answer: A

The muscles in the plantar region of the foot may be divided into three groups, in a similar manner to those in the hand. Those of the medial plantar region are connected with the great toe, and correspond with those of the thumb; those of the lateral plantar region are connected with the little toe, and correspond with those of the little finger; and those of the intermediate plantar region are connected with the tendons intervening between the two former groups. To facilitate the description of these muscles, however, it is more convenient to divide them into four layers, in the order in which they are successively exposed. The first layer contains abductor hallucis, flexor digitorum brevis and abductor digiti minimi. The second layer contains flexor accessorius and lumbricales. The third layer has three muscles, namely flexor hallucis brevis, adductor hallucis and flexor digiti minimi brevis. The fourth layer includes four dorsal and three plantar interossei.

1.31

Answer: B

The oesophagus is closely related to the posterior surface of the pericardial sac. After coming from the heart, the aorta arches over the left pulmonary artery and left bronchus. Eventually, just above the diaphragm, this vessel is posterior to the oesophagus. The azygos vein, on the right side of the thorax, arches over the right pulmonary artery and bronchus. It is also posterior to the oesophagus. The thoracic duct is posterior to the oesophagus as well and does not contact the pericardial sac. Finally, the trachea is superior to the heart.

anatomy

1.32

Answer: C

The median and ulnar nerve both innervate flexor digitorum profundus. Flexor carpi ulnaris is innervated by the ulnar nerve only. Flexor digitorum superficialis and flexor pollicis longus are innervated by the median nerve. Pronator quadratus is innervated by the anterior interosseus nerve, which is a branch of the median nerve.

1.33

Answer: A

The recurrent branch of the median nerve innervates the thenar compartment of the hand, including flexor pollicis brevis, abductor pollicis brevis and opponens pollicis. Therefore, if the median nerve were compressed, all of these muscles could be affected. The dorsal interossei, palmar interossei and opponens digiti minimi are all muscles of the hand that are innervated by the deep branch of the ulnar nerve. Flexor pollicis longus is innervated by the median nerve, but it is a forearm muscle that is proximal to the carpal tunnel, so it would not be affected by compressing the median nerve in the carpal tunnel.

1.34

Answer: B

It is fairly common for the lunate to be dislocated anteriorly; this injury may result from a fall on a dorsiflexed wrist. The lunate may be pushed out of its place on the floor of the carpal tunnel and move towards the palm of the wrist. This dislocation may compress the median nerve and lead to carpal tunnel syndrome. The lateral bone in the proximal row of carpals, which is also scaphoid, is frequently fractured when someone falls on an outstretched wrist. Capitate, hamate and trapezoid are not commonly injured in these falls.

1.35

Answer: E

About 75% of the lymph draining the breast goes to the axillary lymph nodes, via the pectoral lymph nodes. All of this lymph from the pectoral lymph nodes must drain to the central lymph nodes as well. This is why it is so important to examine all these groups of axillary lymph nodes when performing a breast examination. Most of the rest of the lymph drainage from the breast goes to the parasternal nodes, although a small amount goes to the opposite breast and a further small amount drains to the abdominal wall.

1.36

Answer: A

An injury to the long thoracic nerve denervates serratus anterior, meaning that there will be no muscle protracting the scapula and counteracting trapezius and the rhomboids, powerful retractors of the scapula. This means that the scapula will be winged backwards, which is this patient's main symptom. The long thoracic nerve is derived from the nerve roots of C5–C7. This nerve is particularly vulnerable to iatrogenic injury during surgical procedures, such as mastectomies, because it is located on the superficial side of serratus anterior.

The accessory nerve innervates trapezius, so an injury to this nerve might lead to an inability to raise the acromion of the shoulder. The lateral pectoral nerve is a small nerve that provides innervation to pectoralis major. The phrenic nerve innervates the diaphragm. The vagus nerve provides parasympathetic innervation to the thorax and much of the abdominal viscera. The patient's symptoms do not fit with an injury to any of these nerves.

1.37

Answer: B

The artery of Adamkiewicz is also known as the great radicular artery. It is frequently found on the left side in the lower thoracic or upper lumbar region. Similar to all other radicular arteries, it must run with rootlets to reach the spinal cord. The great radicular artery anastomoses on the surface of the thoracic spinal cord and serves as a major blood supply for the lower spinal cord. In fact, disruption of this artery may lead to paraplegia as a result of infarction of the lumbar and sacral portions of the spinal cord. It has a variable origin from level T9 to L3 but has been found to originate as low as L5. Abdominal aortic aneurysm thrombosis can occlude the origin of this artery as can aortic dissection, resulting in acute spinal ischaemia. In all cases of abdominal aorta surgery, preoperative investigations to determine the (variable) origin of the artery of Adamkiewicz are necessary. Identification of its site of origin reduces the incidence of spinal cord injury and surgery time during the repair of thoracoabdominal or descending aorta aneurysms.

1.38

Answer: A

The basilic vein is on the ulnar side of the forearm, near the fifth finger. It arises from the medial side of the dorsal venous arch of the hand and drains blood from the medial (ulnar) side of the arm. The cephalic vein takes its origin from the lateral side of the dorsal venous arch of the hand and then runs up the lateral (radial) forearm. The median antebrachial vein runs down the centre of the anterior forearm, draining into the median cubital vein. The median cubital vein connects the cephalic vein to the basilic vein in the cubital fossa. Finally, the ulnar vein is a deep vein that runs with the ulnar artery.

1.39

Answer: C

The posterior and anterior circumflex arteries wrap around the humerus near its surgical neck. A fracture to the surgical neck could damage either of these arteries or the axillary nerve. The subscapular artery is a branch of the third part of the axillary artery – it branches to form the thoracodorsal artery and the circumflex scapular artery. The radial recurrent artery is a branch of the radial collateral artery; it contributes to collateral circulation around the elbow. The brachial artery is an artery situated deep in the arm; it is close to the humerus, so fracture of the shaft of humerus at midarm might result in damage to this vessel.

1.40

Answer: B

Sustentaculum tali is a shelf-like, medial projection of the calcaneus that supports the talus. The tendon of flexor hallucis longus passes under sustentaculum tali, creating a groove in the bone. So, if sustentaculum tali were fractured, the tendon of flexor hallucis longus would be displaced from its usual position and the muscle would be affected. The peroneus longus tendon enters the foot on the lateral side. It grooves the cuboid bone and travels deep to the long plantar ligament to insert on the medial cuneiform bone. The tendon of flexor digitorum longus crosses on to the plantar surface anterior to sustentaculum tali and eventually divides into four tendons that insert into the bases of the distal phalanges of the second to fifth digits. The tendon from tibialis anterior crosses the dorsal side of the foot and inserts on the medial surface of the first cuneiform and first metatarsal. Finally, the tibialis posterior tendon crosses under the foot on the medial side, anterior to both flexor hallucis longus and flexor digitorum longus. It inserts on navicular, medial cuneiform and second to fourth metatarsals.

1.41

Answer: A

The lateral and medial plantar nerves are both branches of the tibial nerve. These branches continue to the plantar surface of the foot, innervating the muscles there and providing cutaneous innervation to the skin of the sole. The sural nerve is a cutaneous nerve that provides sensory innervation to the skin of the posterior surface of the lower leg and the skin of the lateral side of the foot. The deep peroneal nerve innervates the anterior compartment of the leg and the muscles on the dorsum of the foot, and provides sensory innervation to the web of skin between the first and second toes. The saphenous nerve is a branch of the femoral nerve that travels with the great saphenous vein; it provides cutaneous innervation to the skin of the medial sides of both the leg and the foot. The femoral nerve innervates the anterior (quadriceps) compartment of the thigh, which allows for extension at the knee.

1.42

Answer: E

'Scissor gait' is a condition in which one limb crosses in front of the other during stepping as a result of powerful hip adduction caused by continuous, unwanted, nerve activity. The obturator nerve innervates the medial (adductor) compartment of the thigh, including adductor longus, magnus and brevis. If the obturator nerve were firing too much, the leg would be constantly adducting, causing the scissor gait. The femoral nerve innervates the quadriceps muscles, which extend the leg at the knee. The tibial nerve innervates the hamstrings, which flex the knee and extend the thigh. The tibial nerve also innervates the muscles of the posterior compartment of the leg, which plantarflex the foot. The saphenous nerve is a branch of the femoral nerve that travels with the great saphenous vein; it provides cutaneous innervation to the skin of the medial side of both the leg and the foot. The inferior gluteal nerve innervates gluteus maximus, which is important for powerful extension of the thigh.

1.43

Answer: D

The medial circumflex femoral artery supplies blood to the femoral neck. During fractures of the femoral neck, this artery may be ruptured and the femoral neck deprived of blood. The internal pudendal artery is the major source of blood to the perineum. The perforating branches of the deep femoral artery supply the posterior compartment of the thigh, including the hamstrings. The lateral circumflex femoral artery supplies the lateral thigh and hip. Although it contributes to the circulation around the hip, the primary supply to the head of the femur usually comes from the medial femoral circumflex. The descending genicular artery branches from the femoral artery, just superior to the adductor hiatus, and supplies blood to the knee joint.

1.44

Answer: A

The left gastric artery is the artery that supplies the lesser curvature of the stomach (along with the right gastric artery.) These two arteries would be the most likely to cause bleeding at the lesser curvature of the stomach. The left gastric is one of the three arteries that come off the coeliac trunk. The left and right gastroepiploic arteries are the two arteries that supply the greater curvature of the stomach. The qastroduodenal artery is a branch off the common hepatic artery, which supplies the duodenum, head of pancreas and greater curvature of the stomach. The short gastric arteries are four or five small arteries from the splenic artery that supply the fundus of the stomach.

1.45

Answer: E

The splenorenal ligament is the peritoneal structure that connects the spleen to the posterior abdominal wall over the left kidney. It also contains the tail of the pancreas. The transverse mesocolon connects the transverse colon to the posterior abdominal wall. The gastrocolic ligament connects the greater curvature of the stomach with the transverse colon. The gastrosplenic ligament connects the greater curvature of the stomach with the hilum of the spleen. Finally, the phrenicolic ligament connects the splenic flexure of the colon to the diaphragm.

anatomy

1.46

Answer: B

The spleen is the only organ listed that is covered entirely by visceral peritoneum. The kidney and suprarenal glands are retroperitoneal organs. This is different to the secondarily retroperitoneal organs, which started out in a mesentery and were then pushed against the posterior wall. The kidneys and suprarenal glands began developing in the retroperitoneum and stayed there. The duodenum and pancreas are partially peritonealised and partially retroperitoneal. The first 2 cm of the superior duodenum is peritonealised, but the rest of the duodenum, up to the duodenojejunal junction, is retroperitoneal. For the most part, the pancreas is secondarily retroperitoneal, although the tail of the pancreas is peritonealised, lying within the splenorenal ligament.

1.47

Answer: C

The third, preaortic, transverse or horizontal portion of the duodenum is from 5 to 7.5 cm long. It begins at the right side of the upper border of the fourth lumbar vertebra and passes from right to left, with a slight inclination upwards, in front of the great vessels and crura of the diaphragm; it ends in the ascending portion in front of the abdominal aorta. The superior mesenteric vessels and mesentery cross it and its front surface is covered by peritoneum, except near the middle line where it is crossed by the superior mesenteric vessels. Its posterior surface is not covered by peritoneum, except towards its left extremity, where the posterior layer of the mesentery may sometimes be found covering it to a variable extent. This surface rests on the right crus of the diaphragm, the IVC and the aorta. The upper surface is in relation with the head of the pancreas.

1.48

Answer: D

Compared with the ileum the jejunum is wider, its diameter being about 4 cm, and it is thicker, more vascular and of a deeper colour than the ileum, so that a given length weighs more. The circular folds (valvulae conniventes) of the jejunum's mucous membrane are large and thickly set, and its villi are larger than in the ileum. The aggregated lymph nodules are almost entirely absent in the upper part of the jejunum; in the lower part, they are found less frequently than in the ileum, are smaller and tend to assume a circular form. By grasping the jejunum between the finger and thumb, the circular folds can be felt through the walls of the gut, these being absent in the lower part of the ileum. It is possible in this way to distinguish the upper from the lower part of the small intestine.

1.49

Answer: C

The ileum is narrow, its diameter being 3.75 cm, and its coat thinner and less vascular than that of the jejunum. It possesses just a few circular folds, which are small and disappear entirely towards its lower end, although aggregated lymph nodules (Peyer's patches) are larger and more numerous. For the most part the jejunum occupies the umbilical and left iliac regions, whereas the ileum occupies chiefly the umbilical, hypogastric, right iliac and pelvic regions. The terminal part of the ileum usually lies in the pelvis, from which it ascends over the right psoas and right iliac vessels; it ends in the right iliac fossa by opening into the medial side of the start of the large intestine. The jejunum and ileum are attached to the posterior abdominal wall by an extensive fold of peritoneum, the mesentery, which allows the freest motion, so that each coil can accommodate itself to changes in form and position.

1.50

Answer: D

The head of the pancreas is flattened backwards and lodged within the curve of the duodenum. Its upper border is overlapped by the superior part of the duodenum and its lower border overlaps the horizontal part; its right and left borders overlap in front and insinuate themselves behind the descending and ascending parts of the duodenum, respectively. The greater part of the right half of its anterior surface is in contact with the transverse colon, with only areolar tissue intervening. From its upper part, the neck springs, its right limit being marked by a groove for the gastroduodenal artery. The lower part of the right half, below the transverse colon, is covered by peritoneum continuous with the inferior layer of the transverse mesocolon; this is in contact with the coils of the small intestine. The superior mesenteric artery passes down in front of the left half across the uncinate process; the superior mesenteric vein runs upwards on the right side of the artery and, behind the neck, joins with the splenic vein to form the portal vein. The posterior surface is in relation with the IVC, common bile duct, renal veins, right crus of the diaphragm and aorta.

1.51

Answer: A

The main pancreatic duct, also called the duct of Wirsung, extends transversely from left to right through the substance of the pancreas. It starts by the junction of the small ducts of the lobules, situated in the tail of the pancreas; running from left to right through the body, it receives the ducts of the various lobules that make up the gland. Considerably augmented in size, it reaches the neck and, turning downwards, backwards and to the right, it comes into relation with the common bile duct, which lies to its right side. Leaving the head of the gland, it passes very obliquely through the mucous and muscular coats of the duodenum, ending by an orifice common to it and the common bile duct on the summit of the duodenal papilla, situated at the medial side of the descending (second) portion of the duodenum, 7.5–10 cm below the pylorus. Sometimes, the pancreatic duct and the common bile duct open separately into the duodenum. Frequently, there is an additional duct, which is given off from the pancreatic duct in the neck of the pancreas and opens into the duodenum about 2.5 cm above the duodenal papilla. It receives the ducts from the lower part of the head, and is known as the accessory pancreatic duct (duct of Santorini).

The pancreas is developed in two parts: dorsal and ventral. The former arises as a diverticulum from the dorsal aspect of the duodenum a short distance above the hepatic diverticulum; growing upwards and

ANSWERS

backwards into the dorsal mesogastrium, it forms part of the head and uncinate process and the whole of the body and tail of the pancreas. The ventral part appears in the form of a diverticulum from the primitive bile duct and forms the remainder of the head and uncinate process of the pancreas. The duct of the dorsal part (accessory pancreatic duct) therefore opens independently into the duodenum, whereas that of the ventral part (pancreatic duct) opens with the common bile duct.

1.52

Answer: E

A narrow portion of the anterior surface of the right kidney at the upper extremity is in relation with the right suprarenal gland. A large area just below this, involving about three-quarters of the surface, lies in the renal impression on the inferior surface of the liver, and a narrow but somewhat variable area near the medial border is in contact with the descending part of the duodenum. The lower part of the anterior surface is in contact laterally with the right colic flexure, and medially, as a rule, with the small intestine. The areas in relation with the liver and small intestine are covered by peritoneum; the suprarenal, duodenal and colic areas are devoid of peritoneum. The posterior relations of the right kidney are: the last thoracic, iliohypogastric and ilioinguinal nerves, the diaphragm, medial and lateral lumbocostal arches, psoas major, quadratus lumborum and the tendon of transversus abdominis, the subcostal and one or two of the upper lumbar arteries, as well as the twelfth rib.

1.53

Answer: C

The superior surface of the liver comprises part of both lobes; as a whole, it is convex and fits under the vault of the diaphragm, which in front separates it on the right from the sixth to the tenth ribs and their cartilages, and on the left from the seventh and eighth costal cartilages. Its middle part lies behind the xiphoid process and, in the angle between the diverging rib cartilage of opposite sides, it is in contact with the abdominal wall. Behind this the diaphragm separates the liver from the lower part of the lungs and pleurae, the heart and pericardium, and the right costal arches from the seventh to the eleventh ribs inclusive. It is completely covered by peritoneum, except along the line of attachment of the falciform ligament.

1.54

Answer: D

The oesophagus is a muscular canal, about 23–25 cm (10 inches) long, extending from the pharynx to the stomach. It begins in the neck at the lower border of the cricoid cartilage, opposite the sixth cervical vertebra, descends along the front of the vertebral column, through the superior and posterior mediastina, passes through the diaphragm and, entering the abdomen, ends at the cardiac orifice of the stomach, opposite the eleventh thoracic vertebra. The arteries supplying the oesophagus are derived from the inferior thyroid branch of the thyrocervical trunk, the descending thoracic aorta, the left gastric branch of the coeliac artery and the left inferior phrenic branch of the abdominal aorta. They have for the most part a longitudinal direction. The nerves are derived from the vagi and the sympathetic trunks; they form a plexus, in which there are groups of ganglion cells, between the two layers of the muscular coats, and also a second plexus in the submucous tissue.

1.55

Answer: B

The pudendal nerve is found about 2 cm lateral to the anal canal, so it is the structure most likely to be damaged by the stab wound. The crus of the penis is the lateral part of the corpus cavernosum found at the base of the penis. It is anterior, not lateral, to the anal canal. The perineal body is a structure found in the female only; it is a fibromuscular mass found in the plane between the anal canal and the perineal membrane, which serves at the convergence of several muscles. It is anterior to the anal canal. The inferior rectal artery is a branch of the internal pudendal artery, which delivers blood to the inferior part of the rectum. It would not be injured by the stabbing because it is located on the surface of the rectum, not 2 cm lateral to the anal canal. Finally, the vesicular bulb is a structure of erectile tissue located on either side of the vestibule of the vagina, attached to the perineal membrane, so it would be anterior to the site of the stabbing.

1.56

Answer: F

The prostate is a firm, partly glandular and partly muscular body, which is placed immediately below the internal urethral orifice and around the start of the urethra. It is situated in the pelvic cavity, below the lower part of the symphysis pubis, above the superior fascia of the urogenital diaphragm and in front of the rectum, through which it may be distinctly felt, especially when enlarged. It is about the size of a chestnut and somewhat conical in shape; for examination it presents a base, an apex, and an anterior, a posterior and two lateral surfaces. It is held in its position by the puboprostatic ligaments, the superior fascia of the urogenital diaphragm, which invests the prostate and the start of the membranous portion of the urethra, and the anterior portions of the levator ani muscles, which pass backwards from the pubis and embrace the sides of the prostate. From the support that they afford to the prostate, these portions of the levator ani are named the levator prostatae. The prostate is perforated by the urethra and the ejaculatory ducts. The urethra usually lies along the junction of its anterior with its middle third. The ejaculatory ducts pass obliquely downwards and forwards through the posterior part of the prostate, and open into the prostatic portion of the urethra.

1.57

Answer: C

The ureter measures from 25 to 30 cm in length; it is a thick-walled, narrow, cylindrical tube that is directly continuous near the lower end of the kidney with the tapering extremity of the renal pelvis. It runs downwards and medially in front of the psoas major; entering the pelvic cavity, it finally opens into the fundus of the bladder. At its origin the right ureter is usually covered by the descending part of the duodenum, and in its course downwards lies to the right of the IVC; it is crossed by the right colic and ileocolic vessels, whereas near the superior aperture of the pelvis it passes behind the lower part of the mesentery and the terminal part of the ileum. The left ureter is crossed by the left colic vessels; near the superior aperture of the pelvis it passes behind the sigmoid colon and its mesentery. The arteries supplying the ureter are branches from the renal, internal spermatic, hypogastric and inferior vesical. The nerves are derived from the inferior mesenteric, spermatic and pelvic plexus.

1.58

Answer: D

This is the classic presentation of psoas abscess secondary to tuberculosis (TB) of the spine. TB of the spine forms 50–60% of the total incidence of skeletal TB. It is a disease of childhood and adolescence, 50% of cases occurring before the age of 20. The most common level of the lesion is the thoracolumbar. This is because movement and the stress of weight-bearing are maximum at this level. The proximity of the cysterna chyli may cause lymphatic spread of the infection from foci in the mesenteric lymph glands. The disease affects the spine secondarily from a primary focus in the lungs or mediastinal glands through the bloodstream. The formation of a cold abscess is an invariable feature of TB of the spine. The abscess forms in the paravertebral areas and soon tracks downwards, as a result of gravity, and towards the surface, following the tracks of nerves and blood vessels. As long as the abscess remains deep to the deep fascia, it remains cold to touch with no inflammatory reaction; hence, its name – cold abscess. There is no correlation between the size of the destructive lesion and the quantity of pus in the cold abscess. The size is determined by the degree of allergic exudative reaction that produces the pus. Thoracolumbar cold abscess can either point in the back or enter the psoas sheath and track down as psoas and iliac abscesses. These abscesses collect as lumps in the iliac fossa and point above the inguinal ligament, or track down behind the inguinal ligament and point in the femoral triangle or even lower down. A search for the cold abscess including a careful palpation of the abdomen is an essential part of the clinical examination.

1.59

Answer: B

The transpyloric plane lies halfway between the jugular notch and the upper border of the pubic symphysis. It also lies roughly a hand's breadth below the xiphisternal joint. Anteriorly, it passes through the tip of the ninth costal cartilage. Posteriorly, it passes through the body of the first lumbar vertebra near its lower border. It cuts through the pylorus.

1.60

Answer: C

The popliteal artery is the continuation of the femoral artery, and courses through the popliteal fossa. It extends from the opening in the adductor magnus, at the junction of the middle and lower thirds of the thigh, downwards and laterally to the intercondyloid fossa of the femur, and then vertically downwards to the lower border of the popliteus, where it divides into anterior and posterior tibial arteries. The anterior relations of the artery from above downwards are the popliteal surface of the femur (which is separated from the vessel by some fat), the back of the knee joint and the fascia covering the popliteus. Posteriorly, it is overlapped by semimembranosus above, and covered by gastrocnemius and plantaris below. In the middle part of its course the artery is separated from the skin and fasciae by a quantity of fat, and is crossed from the lateral to the medial side by the tibial nerve and popliteal vein, the vein being between the nerve and the artery and closely adherent to the latter. On its lateral side, above, are biceps femoris, the tibial nerve, the popliteal vein and the lateral condyle of the femur; below are plantaris and the lateral head of gastrocnemius. On its medial side, above, are semimembranosus and the medial condyle of the femur; below are the tibial nerve, the popliteal vein and the medial head of gastrocnemius.

1.61

Answer: D

The facial nerve enters the temporal bone with the vestibulocochlear nerve – both cross into the internal acoustic meatus. The glossopharyngeal (CN IX), vagus (CN X) and spinal accessory (CN XI) nerves all leave through the jugular foramen. The abducent (CN VI) crosses through the superior orbital fissure, along with the oculomotor (CN III), trochlear (CN IV) and ophthalmic division of trigeminal (CN V1) nerves. The three divisions of the trigeminal nerve all leave through different foramina: the ophthalmic division exits through the superior orbital fissure; the maxillary division leaves through the foramen rotundum; and the mandibular division leaves through the foramen ovale.

1.62

Answer: E

The spinal root of the accessory nerve crosses the transverse process of atlas at the C1 level. The superior cervical ganglion is situated at the C2 level. The stellate ganglion is located at the C7 level. The cricoid cartilage corresponds to the C6 level. The C4 vertebral level corresponds to bifurcation of the common carotid arteries as well as the upper border of the thyroid cartilage.

1.63

Answer: A

Technically, the knee joint is regarded as consisting of three articulations in one: two condyloid joints, one between each condyle of the femur and the corresponding meniscus and condyle of the tibia; and a third between the patella and the femur, partly arthrodial, but not completely so, because the articular surfaces are not mutually adapted to each other, so that the movement is not a simple gliding one. The cruciate ligaments are of considerable strength, situated in the middle of the joint, nearer to its posterior than to its anterior surface. They are called cruciate because they cross each other somewhat like the lines of the letter X, and have received the names anterior and posterior, from the position of their attachments to the tibia. The posterior cruciate ligament is stronger, but shorter and less oblique in its direction, than the anterior. The menisci are two crescent-shaped lamellae, which serve to deepen the surfaces of the head of the tibia for articulation with the condyles of the femur. The medial meniscus is almost semicircular in form whereas the lateral meniscus is almost circular and covers a larger portion of the articular surface than the medial one. The ligamentum patellae is the central portion of the common tendon of quadriceps femoris, which is continued from the patella to the tuberosity of the tibia.

1.64

Answer: B

The supraclavicular nerves arise from the third and fourth cervical (C3, C4) nerves; they emerge beneath the posterior border of sternocleidomastoid, and descend in the posterior triangle of the neck beneath platysma and deep cervical fascia. Near the clavicle they perforate the fascia and platysma to become cutaneous, and are arranged, according to their position, into three groups: anterior, middle and posterior. These cutaneous nerves provide sensory innervation to the skin of the root of the neck, upper chest and upper shoulder. These nerves innervate the skin right above the clavicle. The great auricular nerve comes from C2 and C3 branches in the cervical plexus; it provides sensory innervation to the ear and the skin below the ear. The lesser occipital nerve comes from C2 in the cervical plexus – it innervates the skin behind the ear. The transverse cervical nerve is also a cutaneous branch from the cervical plexus – it is from C2 and C3 and provides sensory innervation to the skin of the neck anteriorly. The suprascapular nerve is not a cutaneous nerve – it comes from the superior trunk of the brachial plexus and provides motor innervation to supraspinatus and infraspinatus.

1.65

Answer: E

The superior pancreaticoduodenal artery is a branch of the gastroduodenal artery, which in turn is a branch of the common

anatomy

hepatic artery, itself a branch of the coeliac trunk. The inferior pancreaticoduodenal artery is a branch of the superior mesenteric artery. Occlusion of the coeliac trunk would allow blood from the superior mesenteric artery to reach the branches of the coeliac trunk via the connections between the superior and inferior pancreaticoduodenal arteries. Both the left and right gastric arteries receive their blood from the coeliac trunk. The left gastric artery is a direct branch of the coeliac trunk. The right gastric artery is usually a branch of the proper hepatic artery, which in turn is a branch of the common hepatic artery (a branch of the coeliac trunk). Both the left and right gastroepiploic arteries receive their blood supply from the coeliac trunk. The left gastroepiploic artery is a branch of the splenic artery, which in turn is a branch of the coeliac trunk. The right gastroepiploic artery is a branch of the gastroduodenal artery, which in turn is a branch of the common hepatic artery (a branch of the coeliac trunk). The proper hepatic and gastroduodenal arteries are branches of the common hepatic artery, which in turn is a branch of the coeliac trunk. The right colic and middle colic arteries are both branches of the superior mesenteric artery.

1.66

Answer: C

The anterior continuation of the cavernous sinus, the superior ophthalmic vein, passes through the superior orbital fissure to enter the orbit. Veins of the face communicate with the superior ophthalmic vein. As a result of the absence of valves in emissary veins, venous flow may occur in either direction. Cutaneous infections may be carried into the cavernous sinus and result in a cavernous sinus infection, which may lead to an infected cavernous sinus thrombosis. The cavernous sinus is lateral to the pituitary gland and contains portions of cranial nerves III, IV, V1, V2 and VI, and the internal carotid artery. The occipital sinus is at the base of the falx cerebelli in the posterior cranial fossa. It drains into the confluence of sinuses. The sigmoid sinus is the anterior continuation of the transverse sinus in the middle cranial fossa. The sigmoid sinus passes through the jugular foramen and drains into the internal jugular vein. The straight sinus is at the intersection of the falx cerebri and the falx cerebelli in the posterior cranial fossa. The straight sinus connects the inferior sagittal sinus with the confluence of sinuses. The superior petrosal sinus is at the apex of the petrous portion of the temporal bone and is a posterior continuation of the cavernous sinus. The superior petrosal sinus connects the cavernous sinus with the sigmoid sinus.

1.67

Answer: B

Tumours of the ventricular system of the brain can affect the brain tissue either directly, via pressure on or invasion into a physically close structure, or indirectly, by obstructing cerebrospinal fluid (CSF) flow and causing hydrocephalus. The caudate nucleus is a C-shaped structure that comprises part of the wall of the lateral ventricle throughout its extent. The only structure listed that is adjacent to the body of the lateral ventricle, and would therefore be directly affected by the large tumour arising from the choroidal plexus of the lateral ventricle, is the caudate nucleus. The cerebellum overlies the fourth ventricle. The hippocampus is adjacent to the inferior (temporal) horn of the lateral ventricle; the hypothalamus abuts the third ventricle; the pons forms part of the floor of the fourth ventricle.

1.68

Answer: D

This manoeuvre is meant to test adduction of the index finger and abduction of the middle finger. When testing for abduction and adduction of digits in the hand, it is important to remember that the midline extends through the middle digit. So, this patient is trying to adduct his index finger by pulling it towards the midline and abduct his middle finger by pulling it away from the midline. This means that the patient is using the first palmar interosseous muscle (the adductor) on his index finger and the second dorsal interosseous muscle (the abductor) on his middle finger.

1.69

Answer: A

The epiploic foramen, also called the omental foramen, is the passageway between the greater and lesser peritoneal sacs. The IVC lies immediately posterior to this foramen, so this is the vessel that was probably injured. The aorta lies next to the IVC, but it is a little more to the left and a little deeper; it does not therefore lie immediately posterior to the epiploic foramen. The hepatic portal vein is anterior to the epiploic foramen. The right renal artery is a branch of the aorta. Similar to the aorta, it is too deep to be a vessel immediately behind the foramen. Finally the superior mesenteric vein is anterior to the foramen. As this is one of the two vessels that makes the hepatic portal vein, if the hepatic portal vein is anterior to the foramen, the superior mesenteric vein should also be anterior.

1.70

Answer: E

The 'triangle of Calot' is formed by the cystic duct laterally, the liver superiorly and the common hepatic duct medially. It is an important landmark in this region, because the cystic artery can be found in the triangle of Calot. During cholecystectomy, the cystic artery needs to be ligated. Although the cystic artery usually branches from the right hepatic artery, there is some variation. However, identification of the triangle of Calot can aid in finding the cystic artery, in that triangle, from where it can be traced back to its origin and ligated there.

1.71

Answer: B

The cremaster is a thin muscular layer, composed of a number of fasciculi that arise from the middle of the inguinal ligament, where its fibres are continuous with those of the internal oblique and also occasionally with transversus abdominis. It passes along the lateral side of the spermatic cord, descends with it through the superficial inguinal ring on the front and sides of the cord, and forms a series of loops that differ in thickness and length in different individuals. At the upper part of the cord the loops are short, but they become longer and longer in succession, the longest reaching down as low as the testis, where a few are inserted into tunica vaginalis. These loops are united by areolar tissue, and form a thin covering over the cord and testis, the cremasteric fascia. The fibres ascend along the medial side of the cord, and are inserted by a small pointed tendon into the tubercle and crest of the pubis and the front of the sheath of rectus abdominis.

1.72

Answer: D

The vena caval opening in the diaphragm is situated at about the level of the fibrocartilage between the eighth and ninth thoracic vertebrae. It is quadrilateral in form and placed at the junction of the right and middle leaflets of the central tendon, so that its margins are tendinous. It transmits the IVC, the wall of which is adherent to the margins of the opening, and some branches of the right phrenic nerve. The manubriosternal junction (angle of Louis) is at the level of T4–5 vertebrae. The inferior angle of the scapula is at the T7 level. The medial end of the spine of the scapula is at the T3 level whereas the suprasternal notch corresponds to the T2–3 vertebral level.

1.73

Answer: B

The internal iliac artery supplies the walls and viscera of the pelvis, the buttock, the generative organs and the medial side of the thigh. It is a short, thick vessel, smaller than the external iliac, and about 4 cm in length. It arises at the bifurcation of the common iliac, opposite the lumbosacral articulation, and, passing downwards to the upper margin of the greater sciatic foramen, divides into two large trunks – anterior and posterior. The anterior division gives rise to the superior, middle and inferior vesical arteries, middle rectal artery, obturator artery, internal pudendal artery, inferior gluteal artery, and uterine and vaginal arteries (in females). The posterior division gives rise to the iliolumbar artery, lateral sacral artery and superior gluteal artery.

1.74

Answer: C

The posterior triangle is bounded, in front by the sternocleidomastoid and behind by the anterior margin of trapezius; its base is formed by the middle third of the clavicle and its apex by the occipital bone. The space is crossed, about 2.5 cm above the clavicle, by the inferior belly of omohyoid, which divides it into two triangles: upper or occipital and lower or subclavian.

1.75

Answer: E

The phrenic nerve contains motor and sensory fibres in the proportion of about two to one. It arises chiefly from the fourth cervical nerve, but receives a branch from the third and another from the fifth (the fibres from the fifth occasionally come through the nerve to the subclavius). It descends to the root of the neck, running obliquely across the front of scalenus anterior, and beneath sternocleidomastoid, the inferior belly of the omohyoid, and the transverse cervical and transverse scapular vessels. It next passes in front of the first part of the subclavian artery, between it and the subclavian vein, and, as it enters the thorax, it crosses the internal mammary artery near its origin. Within the thorax, it descends almost vertically in front of the root of the lung and then between the pericardium and the mediastinal pleura, to the diaphragm, where it divides into branches that pierce that muscle and are distributed to its under-surface. In the thorax, it is accompanied by the pericardiacophrenic branch of the internal mammary artery.

1.76

Answer: A

The thoracodorsal nerve, a branch of the posterior cord of the plexus, derives its fibres from the fifth, sixth and seventh cervical nerves; it follows the course of the subscapular artery, along the posterior wall of the axilla to latissimus dorsi, in which it may be traced as far as the lower border of the muscle. Injury to the thoracodorsal nerve will affect latissimus dorsi.

anatomy

1.77

Answer: C

Flexor digitorum brevis, flexor hallucis brevis, abductor hallucis and the first lumbrical are supplied by the medial plantar nerve; all the other muscles in the sole of the foot are supplied by the lateral plantar. The first dorsal interosseous frequently receives an extra filament from the medial branch of the deep peroneal nerve on the dorsum of the foot and the second dorsal interosseous a twig from the lateral branch of the same nerve.

1.78

Answer: D

The portal vein is about 8 cm in length and formed at the level of the second lumbar vertebra by the junction of the superior mesenteric and lienal veins; the union of these veins takes place in front of the IVC and behind the neck of the pancreas. It passes upwards behind the superior part of the duodenum and then ascends in the right border of the lesser omentum to the right extremity of the porta hepatis, where it divides into a right and a left branch, which accompany the corresponding branches of the hepatic artery into the substance of the liver. In the lesser omentum it is placed behind and between the common bile duct and the hepatic artery, the former lying to the right of the latter. It is surrounded by the hepatic plexus of nerves and accompanied by numerous lymphatic vessels and some lymph glands.

1.79

Answer: E

The medial epicondyle, larger and more prominent than the lateral, is directed a little backwards; it gives attachment to the ulnar collateral ligament of the elbow joint, the pronator teres and a common tendon of origin of some of the flexor muscles of the forearm (including palmaris longus, flexor carpi radialis and flexor carpi ulnaris); the ulnar nerve runs in a groove on the back of this epicondyle. Flexor digitorum profundus is situated on the ulnar side of the forearm, immediately beneath the superficial flexors. It arises from the upper three-quarters

anatomy

of the volar and medial surfaces of the body of the ulna, embracing the insertion of brachialis above and extending below to within a short distance of pronator quadratus. It also arises from a depression on the medial side of the coronoid process, by an aponeurosis from the upper three-quarters of the dorsal border of the ulna, in common with flexor and extensor carpi ulnaris, and from the ulnar half of the interosseous membrane.

1.80

Answer: A

The suprascapular nerve arises from the trunk formed by union of the fifth and sixth cervical nerves. It runs laterally beneath trapezius and omohyoid, and enters the supraspinatous fossa through the suprascapular notch, below the superior transverse scapular ligament; it then passes beneath the supraspinatus, and curves around the lateral border of the spine of the scapula to the infraspinatous fossa. In the supraspinatous fossa it gives off two branches to the supraspinatous muscle and an articular filament to the shoulder joint; in the infraspinatous fossa it gives off two branches to the infraspinatous muscle, in addition to some filaments to the shoulder joint and scapula.

1.81

Answer: C

The internal carotid artery supplies the anterior part of the brain, the eye and its appendages, and sends branches to the forehead and nose. Its size, in the adult, is equal to that of the external carotid, although, in the child, it is larger than this vessel. It is remarkable for the number of curvatures that it presents in different parts of its course. In considering the course and relations of this vessel it is usually divided into four portions: cervical, petrous, cavernous and cerebral. In the neck the internal carotid begins at the bifurcation of the common carotid, opposite the upper border of the thyroid cartilage, and runs perpendicularly upwards, in front of the transverse processes of the upper three cervical vertebrae, to the carotid canal in the petrous portion of the temporal bone. It is comparatively superficial at its start, where it is contained in the carotid triangle, and lies behind and lateral to the external carotid, overlapped by the sternocleidomastoid, and covered by the deep fascia, platysma and integument. It then passes beneath the parotid gland, being crossed by the hypoglossal nerve, the digastric and stylohyoid muscles, and the occipital and posterior auricular arteries. Higher up, it is separated from the external carotid by styloglossus and stylopharyngeus, the tip of the styloid process and the stylohyoid ligament, the glossopharyngeal nerve and the pharyngeal branch of the vagus. It is in relation, behind, with longus capitis, the superior cervical ganglion of the sympathetic trunk and the superior laryngeal nerve; laterally, it is in relation with the internal jugular vein and vagus nerve, the nerve lying on a plane posterior to the artery, and medially with the pharynx, superior laryngeal nerve and ascending pharyngeal artery. At the base of the skull the glossopharyngeal, vagus, accessory and hypoglossal nerves lie between the artery and the internal jugular vein.

1.82

Answer: D

The pterygoid plexus is of considerable size and situated between temporalis and the external pterygoid and partly between the external and internal pterygoids. It receives tributaries corresponding with the branches of the internal maxillary artery. Thus, it receives the sphenopalatine, middle meningeal, deep temporal, pterygoid, masseteric, buccinator, alveolar and some palatine veins, and a branch that communicates with the ophthalmic vein through the inferior orbital fissure. The pterygoid venous plexus drains the infratemporal fossa via the maxillary vein. This plexus communicates freely with the anterior facial vein; it also communicates with the cavernous sinus, via branches through the foramen of Vesalius, foramen ovale and foramen lacerum.

1.83

Answer: B

The masseter is a thick, somewhat quadrilateral muscle, consisting of two portions: superficial and deep. The larger superficial portion arises by a thick, tendinous aponeurosis from the zygomatic process of the maxilla, and from the anterior two-thirds of the lower border of the zygomatic arch; its fibres pass downwards and backwards, to be inserted into the angle and lower half of the lateral surface of the ramus of the mandible. The deep portion is much smaller and more muscular in texture; it arises from the posterior third of the lower border and from the whole of the medial surface of the zygomatic arch; its fibres pass downwards and forwards, to be inserted into the upper half of the ramus and the lateral surface of the coronoid process of the mandible. The deep portion of the muscle is partly concealed, in front, by the superficial portion; behind, it is covered by the parotid gland. The fibres of the two portions are continuous at their insertion. The masseter, along with temporalis and the internal pterygoid, raises the mandible against the maxillae with great force. The masseter and the rest of the muscles of mastication are supplied by the mandibular nerve, a division of the trigeminal nerve (CN V).

1.84

Answer: C

The spinal accessory nerve exits from the jugular foramen and runs backward in front of the internal jugular vein in 66.6% of cases and behind it in 33.3%. The nerve then descends obliquely behind the digastric and stylohyoid to the upper part of the sternocleidomastoid; it pierces this muscle and courses obliquely across the posterior triangle of the neck, to end in the deep surface of trapezius. As it traverses the sternocleidomastoid it gives several filaments to the muscle and joins with branches from the second cervical nerve. In the posterior triangle it unites with the second and third cervical nerves, whereas beneath trapezius it forms a plexus with the third and fourth cervical nerves, and from this plexus fibres are distributed to the muscle.

1.85

Answer: E

The gallbladder is a conical or pear-shaped musculomembranous sac, lodged in a fossa on the under-surface of the right lobe of the liver, and extending from near the right extremity of the porta to the anterior border of the organ. It measures from 7 to 10 cm in length, 2.5 cm in breadth at its widest part, and holds from 30 to 35 ml. It is divided into a fundus, body and neck. The fundus, or broad extremity, is directed downwards, forwards and to the right, and projects beyond the anterior border of the liver; the body and neck are directed upwards and backwards to the left. The upper surface of the gallbladder is attached to the liver by connective tissue and vessels. The under-surface is covered by peritoneum, which is reflected on to it from the surface of the liver. Occasionally the whole of the organ is invested by the serous membrane, and is then connected to the liver by a kind of mesentery. The body is in relation, by its upper surface, with the liver, by its under-surface with the start of the transverse colon, and farther back, usually, with the upper end of the descending portion of the duodenum, although sometimes with the superior portion of the duodenum or pyloric end of the stomach. The fundus is completely invested by peritoneum; it is in relation: in front, with the abdominal wall, immediately below the ninth costal cartilage; and behind with the transverse colon. The neck is narrow and curves upon itself like the letter S; at its point of connection with the cystic duct it presents a well-marked constriction. The cystic duct, about 4 cm long, runs backwards, downwards and to the left from the neck of the gallbladder, and joins the hepatic duct to form the common bile duct.

1.86

Answer: A

The hepatic veins start in the substance of the liver, in the terminations of the portal vein and hepatic artery, and are arranged in two groups: upper and lower. The upper group usually consists of three large veins, which converge towards the posterior surface of the liver and open into the IVC, whereas the IVC is situated in the groove on the back part of the liver. The veins of the lower group vary in number and are small in size; they come from the right and caudate lobes. The hepatic veins run singly and are in direct contact with the hepatic tissue. They have no valves.

1.87

Answer: D

The coeliac ganglia (semilunar ganglia) are two large, irregularly shaped masses with the appearance of lymph glands; they are placed one on either side of the midline in front of the crura of the diaphragm close to the suprarenal glands, which on the right side are placed behind the IVC. The upper part of each of these sympathetic ganglia is joined by the preganglionic sympathetic fibres from the greater splanchnic nerve, whereas the lower part, which is segmented off and named the aorticorenal ganglion, receives the lesser splanchnic nerve and gives off the greater part of the renal plexus. The parasympathetic fibres from the vagi traverse these ganglia without synapsing.

1.88

Answer: E

The costodiaphragmatic recess is the lowest extent of the pleural cavity or space. It is the part of the pleural cavity where the costal pleura changes into the diaphragmatic pleura. It is also the area into which a needle is inserted for thoracocentesis or pleural aspiration, and it is found at different levels in different areas of the thorax. At the midclavicular line, the costodiaphragmatic recess is between the sixth and eighth ribs, at the midaxillary line it is between the eighth and tenth, and at the paravertebral line between the tenth and twelfth. So, a needle inserted into the ninth intercostal space in the midaxillary line should enter the costodiaphragmatic recess. The cupola is the part of the pleural cavity that extends above the level of the first rib into the root of the neck. The cardiac notch is a structure on the left lung that separates the lingula below from the upper portion of the superior lobe of left lung. The oblique pericardial sinus is an area of the pericardial cavity located behind the left atrium of the heart. The costomediastinal recess is found where the costal pleura becomes the mediastinal pleura.

1.89

Answer: B

The left recurrent laryngeal nerve is a branch of the vagus that wraps around the aorta, posterior to ductus arteriosus or ligamentum arteriosum. It then travels superiorly to innervate muscles of the larynx. It is important to protect this nerve during surgery. If the left recurrent laryngeal nerve became paralysed, a patient could experience a hoarse voice or even have difficulty breathing as a result of a laryngeal spasm. The thoracic duct is deep in the chest — it travels between the azygos vein and the aorta, posterior to the oesophagus. The accessory hemiazygos vein is a vein on the left side of the body. It drains the posterolateral chest wall and empties blood into the azygos vein. The left internal mammary artery is a branch of the left subclavian artery that supplies blood to the anterior thoracic wall. The left phrenic nerve runs lateral to the vagus nerve and its branches in the thorax; it is not close enough to be damaged by surgery on the ductus arteriosus.

1.90

Answer: A

A direct inguinal hernia is caused by a weakness in the abdominal muscles that prevents a patient from contracting these muscles strongly. The ilioinguinal nerve is important for innervating the muscles of the lower abdominal wall. Normally the falx inguinalis is pulled down to cover the thin area of weak fascia on the posterior wall of the inguinal canal. So, if this nerve were damaged during the appendicectomy, the man might not be able to contract his abdominal muscles and pull the falx inguinalis over the weak fascia. This could have led him to develop the direct inguinal hernia. The subcostal nerve and the ventral primary ramus of T10 innervate muscles, skin and fascia of the upper abdominal wall. These nerves are too superior to affect the inguinal region. The genitofemoral nerve innervates the cremaster muscle. An injury to this nerve would lead to an inability to elevate the testes, but it would not compromise the strength of the abdominal wall.

anatomy

1.91

Answer: E

The nasopharyngeal (auditory) tube is a connection between the nasal portion of the pharynx and the tympanic cavity that allows pressure to equalise on both sides of the tympanic membrane. It is located in the anterior wall of the middle ear and comprises bone at the tympanic end and cartilage on the pharyngeal end. The pharyngeal mucosa is continuous with the lining of the tympanic cavity and mastoid air cells. This allows infectious material to pass to the middle ear and mastoid area. The sacculus is a fluid-filled sac that is part of the balancing apparatus of the ear; it is located in the vestibule of the ear. The cochlea is the organ of hearing that receives, interprets and transmits sound via the vestibulocochlear nerve (CN VIII). The external auditory meatus is the opening in the temporal bone that allows sound waves to reach the tympanic membrane. The internal auditory meatus is the foramen in the temporal bone that allows the vestibulocochlear and facial nerves to pass into the skull at the base of the brain.

1.92

Answer: C

Chorda tympani lies across the ear drum (tympanic membrane), so it is possible that this nerve was injured. Injury to the chorda tympani will result in loss of taste sensation from the anterior two-thirds of the tongue and no secretomotor innervation to the sublingual and submandibular glands. The mandibular nerve is not close to the ear and would not be damaged by the injury. The glossopharyngeal nerve and lesser petrosal nerve are associated with the promontory of the ear, which is on the medial wall of the middle ear. The great auricular branch of the vagus nerve is a small branch of the vagus that supplies afferent sensory innervation to the external acoustic meatus. This nerve is not close to the tympanic membrane.

1.93

Answer: C

The carotid body is innervated by the carotid branch of the glossopharyngeal nerve. It is a small, reddish-brown, ovoid mass that lies on the medial side of the carotid bifurcation, serving as a chemoreceptor that monitors the level of carbon dioxide in the blood. It is similar in structure to the coccygeal body, which is situated on the middle sacral artery.

1.94

Answer: B

The pisiform bone is known by its small size and its presentation of a single articular facet. It is situated on a plane anterior to the other carpal bones and is spheroidal in form. Its dorsal surface presents a smooth, oval facet, for articulation with the triquetral: this facet approaches the superior, but not the inferior, border of the bone. The volar surface is rounded and rough, and gives attachment to the transverse carpal ligament and to flexor carpi ulnaris and abductor digiti minimi. The lateral and medial surfaces are also rough, the former being concave and the latter usually convex.

1.95

Answer: D

The jugular foramen, a large aperture formed in front by the petrous portion of the temporal and behind by the occipital, lies on the base of the skull behind the carotid canal. It is generally larger on the right than on the left side, and may be subdivided into three compartments. The anterior compartment transmits the inferior petrosal sinus, the intermediate the glossopharyngeal, vagus and accessory nerves, and the posterior the transverse sinus and some meningeal branches from the occipital and ascending pharyngeal arteries.

1.96

Answer: D

The clavicle forms the anterior portion of the shoulder girdle. It is a long bone, curved somewhat like the italic letter *f,* and placed almost horizontally at the upper and anterior part of the thorax, immediately above the first rib. It articulates medially with manubrium sterni and laterally with the acromion of the scapula. It presents a double curvature, the convexity being directed forwards at the sternal end and the concavity at the scapular end. Its lateral third is flattened from above downwards, whereas its medial two-thirds has a rounded or prismatic form. The lateral third has two borders: anterior and posterior. The anterior border is concave, thin and rough, and gives attachment to deltoid. The posterior border is convex, rough and thicker than the anterior, and gives attachment to trapezius.

1.97

Answer: E

The lumbricals are four small fleshy fasciculi, associated with the tendons of flexor digitorum profundus. The first and second arise from the radial sides and volar surfaces of the tendons of the index and middle fingers, respectively, the third from the contiguous sides of the tendons of the middle and ring fingers, and the fourth from the contiguous sides of the tendons of the ring and little fingers. Each passes to the radial side of the corresponding finger, and opposite the metacarpophalangeal articulation is inserted into the tendinous expansion of extensor digitorum communis, covering the dorsal aspect of the finger. By virtue of their insertion into the extensor expansion, they assist in extension of the middle and distal phalanges. The two lateral lumbricals are supplied by the sixth and seventh cervical nerves, through the third and fourth digital branches of the median nerve, whereas the two medial lumbricals are supplied by the eighth cervical nerve, through the deep palmar branch of the ulnar nerve. The third lumbrical muscle frequently receives a twig from the median nerve.

1.98

Answer: C

The deltoid ligament connects medial malleolus with talus, navicular and calcaneus. It is on the medial side of the ankle joint, and its role is to prevent the ankle from dislocating when forcibly everted. So, if a foot were strongly everted, the deltoid ligament could tear. The anterior talofibular ligament connects the lateral malleolus with the talus anterolaterally, and the calcaneofibular ligament connects the lateral malleolus with calcaneus. Both of these ligaments contribute to the lateral ligaments of the ankle and can be damaged during forced inversion of the foot. The plantar calcaneonavicular ligament (spring ligament) connects the sustentaculum tali with the plantar surface of the navicular bone. It provides major support for the medial longitudinal arch of the foot. The anterior tibiofibular ligament connects the tibia and fibula, providing support to the distal ends of these bones.

1.99

Answer: B

The rotator cuff holds the head of the humerus in the glenoid cavity of the scapula; supraspinatus is part of the rotator cuff. The four muscles that comprise the rotator cuff all insert on the greater or lesser tubercle of the humerus. Supraspinatus inserts into the upper facet of the greater tubercle of the humerus and the capsule of the shoulder joint. Infraspinatus inserts into the middle facet of the greater tubercle of the humerus and the capsule of the shoulder joint. Teres minor inserts into the lower facet of the greater tubercle of the humerus and the capsule of the shoulder joint. Subscapularis inserts onto the lesser tubercle of the humerus. The other four muscles listed are not parts of the rotator cuff.

anatomy

1.100

Answer: A

The brachial plexus is formed by the union of the anterior divisions of the lower four cervical nerves and the greater part of the anterior division of the first thoracic nerve; the fourth cervical usually gives a branch to the fifth cervical, and the first thoracic frequently receives one from the second thoracic. The plexus extends from the lower part of the side of the neck to the axilla. The branches of distribution of the brachial plexus for description purposes are arranged into two groups, namely those given off above and below the clavicle. The supraclavicular branches include the suprascapular nerve, dorsal scapular nerve, nerve to subclavius, long thoracic nerve and nerve to longus colli and scaleni. The upper subscapular nerve is an infraclavicular branch. The infraclavicular branches are derived from the three cords of the brachial plexus, but the fasciculi of the nerves may be traced through the plexus to the spinal nerves from which they originate. They are as follows: from the lateral cord arise musculocutaneous nerve (C5–7), lateral anterior thoracic nerve (C5–7), lateral head of median nerve (C6, C7), medial anterior thoracic nerve (C6, C7) and medial antebrachial cutaneous nerve (C6, C7); from the medial cord arise the medial brachial cutaneous nerve (C8, T1), ulnar nerve (C8, T1), medial head of median nerve (C8, T1), upper subscapular nerve (C5, C6) and lower subscapular nerve (C5, C6); from the posterior cord arise thoracodorsal nerve (C5–7), axillary nerve (C5, C6) and radial nerve (C5–8, T1).

anatomy

SECTION 2:
PHYSIOLOGY – ANSWERS

2.1

Answer: B

Low levels of glucose in the circulation and substances that inhibit glucose metabolism, such as 2-deoxy-D-glucose, inhibit insulin. Insulin is also inhibited by decreased amounts of fatty acids and amino acids. The actions of somatostatin, sympathetic nervous stimulation and adrenaline (epinephrine) through α-adrenergic receptors are all inhibitory to insulin release. On the other hand, glucose is the principal stimulus for insulin release. Within 10 minutes of eating a meal rich in carbohydrates, especially simple sugars, blood glucose levels rise above 80 mg/dl and this is sufficient to stimulate the release and synthesis of insulin. In general, naturally occurring hexoses and trioses, monosaccharides that can be metabolised, are more potent stimuli of insulin secretion than those that cannot be metabolised, such as mannose. The oral administration of glucose tends to augment the release of insulin because glucose absorption stimulates the secretion of gastrointestinal (GI) hormones that also stimulate insulin secretion. Gastric inhibitory peptide is the most important GI hormone to stimulate insulin release, but gastrin, secretin and cholecystokinin also play a role. Some amino acids stimulate the secretion of insulin. The two most effective are the essential amino acids arginine and lysine. Fatty acids and ketone bodies cause little if any increase in insulin secretion. Glucagon, growth hormone and adrenaline, acting through its β receptor, all stimulate insulin release, as do parasympathetic nervous system stimulation and cyclic adenosine monophosphate (cAMP).

physiology

2.2

Answer: D

There are several mechanisms regulating the release of antidiuretic hormone (ADH), the most important of which are the following:

- Hypovolaemia or decreased plasma volume, as occurs during haemorrhage and dehydration, results in a decrease in atrial pressure. Specialised stretch receptors within the atrial walls and large veins (cardiopulmonary baroreceptors) entering the atria decrease their firing rate when there is a fall in atrial pressure. Afferent nerve fibres from these receptors synapse within the nucleus tractus solitarius of the medulla, which sends fibres to the hypothalamus, a region of the brain that controls ADH release by the posterior pituitary. Atrial receptor firing normally inhibits the release of ADH by the posterior pituitary. With hypovolaemia or decreased central venous pressure, the decreased firing of atrial stretch receptors leads to an increase in ADH release.
- Hypotension, which decreases arterial baroreceptor firing and leads to enhanced sympathetic activity, increases ADH release.
- Hypothalamic osmoreceptors sense extracellular osmolarity and stimulate ADH release when osmolarity rises, as occurs with dehydration.
- Angiotensin II receptors located in a region of the hypothalamus regulate ADH release – an increase in angiotensin II stimulates ADH release.

2.3

Answer: E

The semilunar valves (aortic and pulmonic valves) are closed at the onset of the isovolumetric relaxation phase of the cardiac cycle. As the ventricles continue to relax and intraventricular pressures fall, a point is reached when the total energy of blood within the ventricles is less than the energy of blood in the outflow tracts. When this occurs, the pressure reversal causes the aortic and pulmonic valves to abruptly close (aortic precedes pulmonic), causing the second heart sound (S2). Valve closure is associated with a small backflow of blood into the ventricles and a characteristic notch (incisura or dicrotic notch) in the aortic and pulmonary artery pressure tracings.

2.4

Answer: A

The resistance to sliding flow between fluid layers can lead to irregular flow known as turbulence. The amount of turbulence in a fluid depends on the velocity and general characteristics of the fluid. If the layers of a fluid slide easily over each other, the fluid is said to exhibit laminar flow and has little turbulence. If the velocity is high enough, the local flow of the fluid may include circular currents that impede the sliding of the layers of the fluid. Reynold's number is a quantity that serves as an indicator for the type of flow that a fluid will exhibit. This number, N_R, depends on the viscosity η, the density ρ, the velocity v and the diameter D of the tube:

$$N_R = \frac{\rho \, v \, D}{\eta}$$

Increasing the length of the vessel may indirectly decrease the likelihood of turbulence by increasing vascular resistance and thus decreasing blood velocity.

2.5

Answer: E

The oxyhaemoglobin dissociation curve is capable of shifting to the right or the left. An increase in the blood P_{CO_2} or hydrogen ion concentration $[H^+]$ (decreased pH) shifts the curve to the right, whereas a decrease in P_{CO_2} or $[H^+]$ (increased pH) shifts the curve to the left. Shifts in the oxyhaemoglobin dissociation curve as a result of changes in the blood P_{CO_2} or pH are termed the Bohr effect. An increase in blood temperature or 2,3-diphosphoglycerate (2,3-DPG) levels in the red blood cells (RBCs) also shifts the oxyhaemoglobin dissociation curve to the right, whereas a decrease in temperature or 2,3-DPG shifts the curve to the left. A shift in the oxyhaemoglobin

physiology

dissociation curve to the right means that more O_2 is liberated for a given decrease in the Po_2.

Stated another way, a shift in the curve to the right indicates that the affinity of haemoglobin for O_2 is reduced, so that, for a given plasma Po_2, more O_2 is freed from the haemoglobin. In contrast, a shift in the curve to the left means that more O_2 will be attached to haemoglobin (increased affinity) for a given $Po2$. Thus, less O_2 is available to the tissues or is freed from haemoglobin at a given Po_2.

2.6

Answer: D

Persistent diarrhoea will result in metabolic acidosis (increase in the H^+ concentration) as a result of the loss of bicarbonate-rich secretions from the pancreas and gallbladder. The response of the body to an increase in the H^+ concentration involves several processes. The first and most readily available process is extracellular buffering. The most readily measured extracellular buffer is carbonic acid (H_2CO_3). This buffer is considered an open buffering system because compensatory mechanisms in respiratory carbon dioxide (CO_2) (increase or decrease in ventilation) and renal HCO_3^- (increase or decrease in kidney reclamation of HCO_3^-) serve to maintain equilibrium. Metabolic acidosis most commonly stimulates the central and peripheral chemoreceptors that control respiration, resulting in an increase in alveolar ventilation, which in turn results in a compensatory respiratory alkalosis. As a result of buffering of H^+ by HCO_3^- the plasma concentration of HCO_3^- will decrease, which will decrease the amount of HCO_3^- that is filtered in the proximal tubule. At the same time, the metabolic acidosis will increase ammonia production by the proximal tubule as well as H^+ secretion and production of new bicarbonate by the distal nephron. As the metabolic acidosis is produced by the loss of bicarbonate, the anion gap will remain within normal limits.

2.7

Answer: B

Haemorrhage is compensated for by several methods that are both acute and chronic fixes for the problem. Rapid compensation for low blood volume include vaso- and venoconstriction, increased heart rate (tachycardia), adrenergic output from the adrenal medulla and sympathetic nerves, secretion of vasopressin, glucocorticoids, renin, aldosterone and erythropoietin, and hepatic plasma protein synthesis. By decreasing urine formation, retaining sodium and water, increasing blood pressure, stimulation of blood cell formation and increasing plasma oncotic pressure, the net effect is to feed the brain and heart while restoring normal blood volume.

2.8

Answer: D

Peristalsis is a distinctive pattern of smooth muscle contractions that propels foodstuffs distally through the oesophagus and intestines. It was first described by Bayliss and Starling as a type of motility in which there is contraction above and relaxation below a segment that is being stimulated. Peristalsis is not affected to any degree by vagotomy or sympathectomy, indicating its mediation by the intestine's local, intrinsic nervous system. Peristalsis is a manifestation of two major reflexes within the enteric nervous system that are stimulated by a bolus of foodstuff in the lumen. Mechanical distension and perhaps mucosal irritation stimulate afferent enteric neurons. These sensory neurons synapse with two sets of cholinergic interneurons, which lead to two distinct effects:

- One group of interneurons activates excitatory motor neurons above the bolus; these neurons, which contain acetylcholine and substance P, stimulate *contraction of smooth muscle above the bolus.*
- Another group of interneurons activates inhibitory motor neurons that *stimulate relaxation of smooth muscle below the bolus.* These inhibitor neurons appear to use nitric oxide, vasoactive intestinal peptide (VIP) and ATP as neurotransmitters.

2.9

Answer: D

Secretin is a peptide hormone made of 27 amino acids, produced in the crypts of Lieberkühn of the duodenum and released in response to a luminal pH < 4.5. It stimulates fluid and bicarbonate release from the pancreas and stimulates pepsinogen secretion.

2.10

Answer: E

Acute respiratory consequences of pulmonary embolism include increased alveolar dead space, pneumoconstriction, hypoxaemia and hyperventilation, leading to low P_{CO_2}. Later, two additional consequences may occur: regional loss of surfactant and pulmonary infarction. Arterial hypoxaemia is a frequent but not universal finding in patients with acute embolism. The mechanisms of hypoxaemia include ventilation/perfusion mismatch, intrapulmonary shunts, reduced cardiac output and intracardiac shunt via a patent foramen ovale. Pulmonary infarction is an uncommon consequence because of the bronchial arterial collateral circulation. Pulmonary embolism reduces the cross-sectional area of the pulmonary vascular bed, resulting in an increment in pulmonary vascular resistance, which, in turn, increases the right ventricular afterload. If the afterload is increased severely, right ventricular failure may ensue. In addition, the humoral and reflex mechanisms contribute to the pulmonary arterial constriction. Prior poor cardiopulmonary status of the patient is an important factor, leading to haemodynamic collapse.

2.11

Answer: A

Starling's hypothesis states that the fluid movement as a result of filtration across the wall of a capillary is dependent on the balance between the hydrostatic pressure gradient and the oncotic pressure gradient across the capillary. The four Starling's forces are:

physiology

1. Hydrostatic pressure in the capillary (P_c)
2. Hydrostatic pressure in the interstitium (P_i)
3. Oncotic pressure in the capillary (π_c)
4. Oncotic pressure in the interstitium (π_i).

The balance of these forces allows calculation of the net driving pressure for filtration:

-   Net driving pressure = $[(P_c - P_i) - (\pi_c - \pi_i)]$

The net fluid flux is proportional to this net driving pressure. To derive an equation to measure this fluid flux several additional factors need to be considered, including:

-   The reflection coefficient
-   The filtration coefficient (K_f).

An additional point to note here is that the capillary hydrostatic pressure falls along the capillary from the arteriolar to the venous end and the driving pressure will decrease (and typically become negative) along the length of the capillary. The other Starling's forces remain constant along the capillary.

The reflection coefficient can be thought of as a correction factor that is applied to the measured oncotic pressure gradient across the capillary wall. Consider the following. The small leakage of proteins across the capillary membrane has two important effects:

1. The interstitial fluid oncotic pressure is higher then it would otherwise be.
2. Not all of the protein present is effective in retaining water so the effective capillary oncotic pressure is lower than the measured oncotic pressure (in the same way that there is a difference between osmolality and tonicity).

Both these effects decrease the oncotic pressure gradient. The interstitial oncotic pressure is accounted for because its value is included in the calculation of the gradient.

The reflection coefficient is used to correct the magnitude of the measured gradient to take account of the 'effective oncotic pressure'. It can have a value from 0 to 1. For example, CSF and the glomerular filtrate have very low protein concentrations and the

physiology

reflection coefficient for protein in these capillaries is close to 1. Proteins cross the walls of the hepatic sinusoids relatively easily and the protein concentration of hepatic lymph is very high. The reflection coefficient for protein in the sinusoids is low. The reflection coefficient in the pulmonary capillaries is intermediate in value: about 0.5.

The net fluid flux (caused by filtration) across the capillary wall is proportional to the net driving pressure. The filtration coefficient is the constant of proportionality in the flux equation (Starling's equation). The filtration coefficient consists of two components because the net fluid flux is dependent on:

1. The area of the capillary walls where the transfer occurs
2. The permeability of the capillary wall to water (this permeability factor is usually considered in terms of the 'hydraulic conductivity' of the wall).

The filtration coefficient is the product of these two components:

- K_f = Area × Hydraulic conductivity
- A 'leaky' capillary (eg as a result of histamine) would have a high filtration coefficient. The glomerular capillaries are naturally very leaky because this is necessary for their function; they have a high filtration coefficient.

Now, using Starling's equation:

Net fluid flux = K_f × (Net driving pressure)

Net fluid flux = $K_f \times [(P_c - P_i) - r_c (\pi_c - \pi_i)]$

where r_c is the reflection coefficient; substituting the values in the question into the equation and solving for interstitial oncotic pressure (π_i) we get:

8 mmHg = 1 × [(24 − 7) −1 × (17 − π_i)]

π_i = 8 mmHg

2.12

Answer: D

Pneumothorax is the presence of air within the pleural space. Pneumothorax is considered to be one of the most common forms of thoracic disease and is classified as spontaneous (not caused by trauma), traumatic or iatrogenic. Entry of air into the pleural space results in collapse of the lung. The primary physical sign of pneumothorax is a decrease or absence of breath sounds despite normal or increased resonance on percussion. However, this may be difficult to detect, particularly in patients with a small pneumothorax or in those who have underlying emphysema. Patients with a small pneumothorax (involving < 15% of the hemithorax) may have a normal physical examination. Tachycardia is the most common physical finding. Large pneumothoraces can cause decreased movement of the chest wall, a hyperresonant percussion note, diminished tactile focal fremitus and resonance, and decreased or absent breath sounds on the affected side. Haemodynamic instability, which is indicated by tachycardia, hypotension and cyanosis, suggests a tension pneumothorax. Arterial blood gases may reveal acute respiratory alkalosis and an increased alveolar–arterial oxygen gradient. Unusual clinical manifestations of pneumothorax include ptosis (as a result of extension of subcutaneous emphysema), pneumocephalus (secondary to tension pneumothorax associated with a comminuted fracture of the thoracic spine) and recurrent pneumopericardium (in association with a pleuropericardial defect).

2.13

Answer: C

As a result of obstruction to venous return, the right atrial pressure falls, leading to a fall in left atrial pressure, which in turn results in a decreased preload on the left ventricle. This decrease in preload lowers cardiac output. The fall in cardiac output is compensated for by an increase in total peripheral resistance, a rise in systemic arterial blood pressure, a fall in the urine production and a rise in the heart rate.

physiology

2.14

Answer: D

Each of these stresses involves obstruction of blood flow into the right atrium. The excess blood in the circulation is pooled in the venous system resulting in engorged veins. Urine production falls, exacerbating the patient's illness. The increase in intravascular pressure causes fluid to be filtered out of the circulation and into the extravascular space, leading to systemic oedema and ascites.

2.15

Answer: B

Voltage-gated sodium channels are crucial for the propagation of action potentials in excitable membranes. They cause the cell membrane to depolarise by allowing the influx of Na^+ into the cell. They have been known to cause this effect for almost half a century. Some 7000 sodium ions pass through each channel during the brief period (about 1 ms) that it remains open. Voltage-gated Na^+ channels consist of an α subunit responsible for selectivity and voltage gating. However, some sodium channels also have one or two smaller subunits called β-1 and β-2. The protein has four homologous domains containing multiple potential α-helical transmembrane segments. The segments are connected by non-conserved, hydrophilic, intervening segments. The fourth transmembrane segment (S4) of each domain is highly positively charged and thought to be a voltage sensor.

2.16

Answer: C

Cells within the sinoatrial (SA) node are the primary pacemaker site within the heart. These cells are characterised as having no true resting potential, but instead generate regular, spontaneous action potentials. Unlike most other cells that elicit action potentials (eg nerve cells, muscle cells), the depolarising current is carried primarily by relatively slow, inward Ca^{2+} currents instead of by fast Na^+ currents. There are, in fact, no fast Na^+ currents operating in SA nodal cells.

physiology

Phase 0 depolarisation is primarily a result of increased Ca^{2+} conductance. As a result of the movement (or conductance) of Ca^{2+} through their channels not being rapid (hence, the term 'slow inward Ca^{2+} channels'), the rate of depolarisation (slope of phase 0) is much slower than found in other cardiac cells (eg Purkinje cells).

2.17

Answer: C

The normal bone marrow examination findings include:

- Fat:cell ratio
- Child aged < 10 years: 10% fat:90% cells
- Adult: 30−70% fat:70−30% cells
- Myeloid:erythroid ratio: 3:1
- Erythroid cells: 18−39% of marrow nucleated cells
- Megakaryocytes: 0.5−2% of nucleated cells in marrow
- Lymphocytes: 11−23% of nucleated cells in marrow
- T lymphocytes: B lymphocytes = 3:1
- Plasma cells: 0.4−3.9% of nucleated cells in marrow
- Myeloid cells: 60−75% of nucleated cells in marrow
- Neutrophilic series: 49−65%
- Eosinophilic series: 1.2−5.3%
- Basophilic series and mast cells: < 0.2%.

2.18

Answer: E

The oil/water partition coefficient (β) is obtained by:

$$[Solute]_{oil}/[Solute]_{water}$$

after dissolving it in a 50:50 oil:water mix. Lipid-soluble compounds (hydrophobic) have high partition coefficients; water-soluble compounds have low partition coefficients.

Molecules with a large β value have a greater effective transmembrane solute gradient for a given concentration difference between the extracellular fluid and cytoplasm. Molecules with a small β value have a lower effective transmembrane solute gradient. Carbon dioxide, steroid hormones and oxygen have high coefficients and hence readily permeate cell membranes.

2.19

Answer: D

Ventricular stroke volume (SV) is the difference between the ventricular end-diastolic volume (EDV) and the end-systolic volume (ESV). In a typical adult heart, the EDV is about 120 ml blood and the ESV about 50 ml blood. The difference in these two volumes, 70 ml, represents the SV. Therefore, any factor that alters either the EDV or the ESV will change the SV:

SV = EDV − ESV

There are three primary mechanisms that regulate EDV and ESV, and therefore SV. SV is regulated is by the Frank–Starling mechanism. Briefly, an increase in preload exemplified by an increase in venous return to the heart increases the ventricular EDV and the force of ventricular contraction, which enables the heart to eject the additional blood that was returned to it. Conversely, a decrease in venous return leads to a decrease in SV by this mechanism. Changes in afterload affect the ability of the ventricle to eject blood and thereby alter ESV and SV. For example, an increase in afterload (eg increased aortic pressure) decreases SV by increasing ESV. Conversely, a decrease in afterload augments SV. Changes in inotropy (contractility) alter the rate of ventricular pressure development thereby affecting ESV and SV. For example, an increase in inotropy (eg sympathetic activation of the heart) decreases ESV and increases SV. Conversely, a decrease in inotropy (eg heart failure) reduces SV by increasing ESV.

2.20

Answer: E

Electrolyte concentration of body fluids

Electrolyte	Plasma (mmol/l)	Interstitial fluid (mmol/l)	Intracellular fluid (mmol/l)
Cations			
Na^+	142	144	10
K^+	4	4	150
Ca^{2+}	2.5	1.5	2
Mg^{2+}	1.5	0.5	20
Anions			
Cl^-	103	114	10
HCO_3^-	27	30	10
SO_4^{2-}	1.5	1.5	70
PO_4^{3-}	1	1	45

2.21

Answer: E

Metabolic acidosis results from the accumulation of non-volatile acids, reduction of renal acid excretion or loss of alkali. Anion gap (normal 3–11 mmol/l) represents those anions, other than Cl^- and HCO_3^-, necessary to counterbalance Na^+ electrically:

Anion gap (AG) (mmol/l) = Na^+ (mmol/l) – Cl^- (mmol/l) + HCO_3^- (mmol/l).

A normal anion gap (hyperchloraemic) metabolic acidosis results from the loss of bicarbonate-rich fluids from the GI tract (eg diarrhoea or pancreatic or biliary fistula) or kidney (eg renal tubular acidosis, K^+-sparing diuretics, carbonic anhydrase inhibitors). It may also occur after the administration of HCl or its precursor (eg in parenteral nutrition) and ureterosigmoidostomy. Increased AG metabolic acidosis occurs in the setting of toxic ingestions (eg salicylates, methanol, ethylene glycol), rhabdomyolysis, overproduction of endogenous acids (eg lactic acidosis, ketoacidosis) or as a consequence of renal failure. Lactic acidosis (normal serum lactate 0.3–1.3 mmol/l) represents one of the most common causes of severe metabolic acidosis encountered in the critically ill surgical patient.

2.22

Answer: A

Although the cause of metabolic alkalosis is usually apparent in the surgical patient, measurement of urinary Cl^- concentration may be useful in differentiating these disorders. Urine Cl^- concentration < 15 mmol/l suggests vomiting, nasogastric suctioning, post-diuretic administration or post-hypercapnia as the cause of the metabolic alkalosis. Urine Cl^- concentration > 20 mmol/l suggests mineralocorticoid excess, alkali loading, concurrent diuretic administration or the presence of severe hypokalaemia.

2.23

Answer: D

Ejection fraction (EF) is the fraction of blood ejected by the ventricle relative to its end-diastolic volume. Therefore, EF is calculated from:

$$EF = (SV/EDV) \times 100$$

where SV is the stroke volume and EDV is the end-diastolic volume.

EF is most commonly measured using echocardiography. This non-invasive technique provides good estimates of EDV, ESV and SV (SV = EDV − ESV).

Normally, EF is > 60%. For example, if the SV is 75 ml and the EDV 120 ml, then the EF is 63%. During exercise in highly conditioned individuals, the increased SV (caused primarily by increased inotropy) can result in the EF exceeding 90%. In heart failure, particularly in dilated cardiomyopathy, the EF can become very small as the SV decreases and EDV increases. In severe heart failure, the EF may be only 20%. The EF is often used as a clinical index to evaluate the inotropic status of the heart. However, it is important to note that there are circumstances in which the EF can be normal, yet the ventricle is in failure. One example is diastolic dysfunction caused by hypertrophy, in which filling is impaired because of low ventricular compliance and SV is therefore reduced.

2.24

Answer: E

This patient has got excess ADH (vasopressin) release, resulting in the syndrome of inappropriate ADH secretion (SIADH). Ordinarily, release of ADH from the posterior pituitary gland occurs as a physiological response to a drop in plasma volume or an increase in serum osmolality. Non-osmotically driven secretion of ADH in the absence of a haemodynamic disturbance characterises SIADH. Specific diagnostic criteria that define SIADH include the following:

- Hyponatraemia (serum Na^+ < 135 mmol/l)
- Hypotonicity (plasma osmolality < 280 mosmol/kg)
- Inappropriately concentrated urine (> 100 mosmol/kg water)

physiology

- Elevated urine Na^+ concentration (> 20 mmol/l), except during Na^+ restriction
- Clinical euvolaemia
- Normal renal, adrenal and thyroid function.

Sodium serves as the major determinant of serum osmolality and reflects the relative ratio of Na^+:H_2O in the blood. ADH, a water-retaining hormone, promotes water retention by increasing the permeability of nephrons. Elevation in the ADH level despite low serum Na^+ levels and decreased osmolality indicates the presence of a non-osmotic stimulus for ADH release. Excess ADH may emerge from the pituitary gland or an ectopic source, such as neoplasms and/or pulmonary tissue.

Neoplastic cells obtained from tumours of patients with SIADH are characterised by the potential to synthesise, store and secrete ADH (eg increased levels of ADH found in about 60% of patients with small cell carcinoma of the lung). Even though hyponatraemia accompanying SIADH arises from an increase in total body water, this condition is sometimes referred to, confusingly, as a cause of euvolaemic hyponatraemia. Patients with SIADH demonstrate relatively normal Na^+ excretion (if intake is normal), high urine osmolality and only subtle evidence of volume expansion.

As most excess body water accumulates intracellularly and not in the intravascular space, evidence of oedema, ascites and heart failure is absent. However, intracellular oedema alters cell functions, with the central nervous system being the most sensitive to these changes.

2.25

Answer: B

This patient had respiratory acidosis as the $Paco_2$ is high and standard bicarbonate is slightly elevated. This is a common finding in acute exacerbations of chronic obstructive pulmonary disease. Respiratory acidosis is a clinical disturbance that is due to alveolar hypoventilation. Production of carbon dioxide occurs rapidly, and failure of ventilation promptly increases the partial arterial pressure of carbon dioxide ($Paco_2$). The reference range for $Paco_2$ is 36−44

physiology

mmHg (4.4–5.9 kPa). Alveolar hypoventilation leads to an increased $Paco_2$ (ie, hypercapnia). The increase in $Paco_2$ in turn decreases the $HCO_3^-/Paco_2$ and decreases pH. Hypercapnia and respiratory acidosis occur when impairment in ventilation occurs and the removal of CO_2 by the lungs is less than the production of CO_2 in the tissues. In acute respiratory acidosis, compensation occurs in two steps. The initial response is cellular buffering that occurs over minutes to hours. Cellular buffering elevates plasma bicarbonate (HCO_3^-) only slightly, approximately 1 mEq/l (1 mmol/l) for each 10 mmHg (1.33 kPa) increase in $Paco_2$. The second step is renal compensation that occurs over 3–5 days. With renal compensation, renal excretion of carbonic acid is increased and bicarbonate reabsorption is increased. In renal compensation, plasma bicarbonate rises 3.5 mEq/l (3.5 mmol/l) for each increase of 10 mmHg (1.33 kPa) in $Paco_2$. The expected change in serum bicarbonate concentration in respiratory acidosis can be estimated as follows:

- Acute respiratory acidosis: HCO_3^- increases 1 mEq/L (1 mmol/l) for each 10-mmHg (1.33 kPa) rise in $Paco_2$
- Chronic respiratory acidosis: HCO_3^- rises 3.5 mEq/L (3.5 mmol/L) for each 10 mmHg (1.33 kPa) rise in $Paco_2$

The expected change in pH with respiratory acidosis can be estimated with the following equations:

- Acute respiratory acidosis:
  Change in pH: $0.008 \times (40 - Paco_2)$
- Chronic respiratory acidosis:
  Change in pH: $0.003 \times (40 - Paco_2)$

Respiratory acidosis does not have a great effect on electrolyte levels. Some small effects occur on calcium and potassium levels. Acidosis decreases binding of calcium to albumin and tends to increase serum ionized calcium levels. In addition, acidaemia causes an extracellular shift of potassium, but respiratory acidosis rarely causes clinically significant hyperkalaemia.

physiology

2.26

Answer: C

The flow-directed balloon-tipped pulmonary artery catheter (also known as the Swan–Ganz catheter) has been in clinical use for almost 30 years. Initially developed for the management of acute myocardial infarction, it now has widespread use in the management of a variety of critical illnesses and surgical procedures. It is used for estimation of pressure in the right atrium (central venous pressure or CVP), right ventricle and pulmonary artery, and of pulmonary artery wedge pressure (PAWP). Other important information provided by a Swan–Ganz catheter includes the cardiac output (CO), mixed venous oxygen saturation Svo_2 and oxygen saturations in the right heart chambers to assess for the presence of an intracardiac shunt. Using these measurements, other variables can be derived, including pulmonary or systemic vascular resistance and the difference between arterial and venous oxygen content.

Systemic vascular resistance (SVR) can be calculated by using the following formula:

$$SVR = (MAP - CVP/CO) \times 80$$

where MAP is the mean arterial pressure.

Thus, substituting the values in this equation, the SVR for this patient is 1440 dyn/cm^2.

2.27

Answer: E

The measurement of the PAWP, also known as the pulmonary capillary wedge pressure (PCWP), provides an indirect measure of left atrial pressure and is particularly useful in the diagnosis of left ventricular failure and mitral stenosis. The measurement is made as follows. A balloon-tipped, multi-lumen (Swan–Ganz) catheter is advanced from a peripheral vein into the right atrium and right ventricle and then positioned within a branch of the pulmonary artery. There is one opening (port) at the tip of the catheter (distal to the balloon) and a second port several centimetres proximal to the balloon. These

physiology

ports are connected to pressure transducers. When properly positioned in a branch of the pulmonary artery, the distal port measures pulmonary artery pressure (about 30/15 mmHg) and the proximal port measures right atrial pressure (about 0–2 mmHg). The balloon is then inflated with air using a syringe (the balloon volume is about 1 ml) which occludes the branch of the pulmonary artery. When this occurs, the pressure in the distal port rapidly falls and, after about 10 seconds, reaches a stable lower value that is very similar to left atrial pressure (normally about 8–10 mmHg). The balloon is then deflated. The recorded pressure during balloon inflation is similar to the left atrial pressure because the occluded vessel, along with its distal branches that eventually form the pulmonary veins, acts as a long catheter that measures the blood pressures within the pulmonary veins (this pressure is virtually the same as mean left atrial pressure). A PAWP exceeding 15 mmHg suggests mitral stenosis, mitral regurgitation, severe aortic stenosis or left ventricular failure. When the PAWP exceeds 20 mmHg, the transmission of this pressure back into the pulmonary vasculature increases pulmonary capillary hydrostatic pressure, which can lead to pulmonary congestion and oedema.

2.28

Answer: A

The parietal cells of the stomach produce intrinsic factor, a glycoprotein that forms a complex with dietary vitamin B_{12}. The stimulus for production can be either vagal, gastrin or histamine signals. The ileum has specific receptors on its enterocytes for the complex. In the presence of calcium ions and a low pH, vitamin B_{12} is then taken up by the cell and intrinsic factor is re-released into the gut. Patients without a stomach and those with pernicious anaemia require injectable vitamin B_{12} replacement therapy. Parietal cells also synthesise and secrete hydrochloric acid. Chief cells secrete pepsinogen, the proenzyme form of pepsin. G-cells secrete gastrin, which stimulates secretion of acid by parietal cells found in the body and fundus of the stomach. Goblet cells are part of the mucosa of the small intestine, not the stomach. Mucus neck cells secrete mucus and are located in the necks of the gastric glands.

physiology

2.29

Answer: B

ADH increases the water permeability of the cortical and medullary collecting tubules and ducts, and allows the filtrate to reach osmotic equilibrium with the interstitial fluid surrounding the nephron. The interstitial fluid in the cortex of the kidney is isotonic to plasma, and therefore the filtrate can become isotonic to plasma in the cortical collecting tubule. The interstitial fluid is hypertonic to plasma in the medullary collecting tubule, and so the filtrate becomes hypertonic to plasma in this region of the nephron and remains hypertonic as it passes through the renal pelvis. ADH has no effect on the water permeability of the loop of Henle. The filtrate is hypertonic to plasma in the descending limb and becomes hypotonic to plasma by the time it reaches the ascending limb of the loop of Henle.

2.30

Answer: D

The patient in this clinical scenario is in haemorrhagic shock as a result of acute external blood loss. The human body responds to acute haemorrhage by activating four major physiological systems: the haematological, cardiovascular, renal and neuroendocrine systems.

The haematological system responds to an acute severe blood loss by activating the coagulation cascade and contracting the bleeding vessels (by means of local thromboxane A_2 release). In addition, platelets are activated (also by means of local thromboxane A_2 release) and form an immature clot on the bleeding source. The damaged vessel exposes collagen, which subsequently causes fibrin deposition and stabilisation of the clot. About 24 h are needed for complete clot fibrination and mature formation.

The cardiovascular system initially responds to hypovolaemic shock by increasing the heart rate, increasing myocardial contractility and constricting peripheral blood vessels. This response occurs secondary to an increased release of noradrenaline (norepinephrine) and decreased baseline vagal tone (regulated by the baroreceptors in the carotid arch, aortic arch, left atrium and pulmonary vessels). The cardiovascular system also responds by redistributing blood to the brain, heart and kidneys and away from the skin, muscle and GI tract.

The renal system responds to haemorrhagic shock by stimulating an increase in renin secretion from the juxtaglomerular apparatus. Renin converts angiotensinogen to angiotensin I, which subsequently is converted to angiotensin II by the lungs and liver. Angiotensin II has two main effects, both of which help to reverse haemorrhagic shock: vasoconstriction of arteriolar smooth muscle and stimulation of aldosterone secretion by the adrenal cortex. Aldosterone is responsible for active sodium reabsorption and subsequent water conservation.

The neuroendocrine system responds to haemorrhagic shock by causing an increase in circulating ADH. ADH is released from the posterior pituitary gland in response to a decrease in blood pressure (as detected by baroreceptors) and a decrease in the sodium concentration (as detected by osmoreceptors). ADH indirectly leads to an increased reabsorption of water and sodium by the distal tubule, collecting ducts and loop of Henle.

2.31

Answer: C

Mitral stenosis is a narrowing of the inlet valve into the left ventricle that prevents proper opening during diastolic filling. Patients with mitral stenosis typically have mitral valve leaflets that are thickened, commissures that are fused and/or chordae tendineae that are thickened and shortened. The most common cause of mitral stenosis is rheumatic fever. About 40% of patients with rheumatic heart disease have isolated mitral stenosis. The normal area of the mitral valve orifice is 4–6 cm^2, which effectively creates a common chamber between the left atrium and the left ventricle in diastole. In early diastole, a small and brief pressure gradient is present, but, during most of the filling period, the pressures in the two chambers are equal. Narrowing of the valve area to less than 2.5 cm^2 impedes the free flow of blood and causes a build-up of left atrial pressure (LAP) to promote normal transmitral flow volume.

physiology

Critical mitral stenosis occurs when the opening is reduced to 1 cm^2. At this stage, an LAP of 25 mmHg is required to maintain a normal cardiac output. With progressive stenosis, critical flow restriction reduces left ventricular output. The increase in LAP also enlarges the left atrium and raises pulmonary venous and capillary pressures. The resulting pulmonary congestion and reduced cardiac output can mimic primary left ventricular failure, but left ventricular contractility is normal in most cases of mitral stenosis. As the disease evolves, chronic elevation of LAP eventually leads to pulmonary hypertension, tricuspid and pulmonary valve incompetence, and secondary right heart failure.

2.32

Answer: B

Sinus bradycardia can be defined as a sinus rhythm with a resting heart rate of 60 beats/min or less. However, few patients actually become symptomatic until their heart rate drops to less than 50 beats/min. The action potential responsible for this rhythm arises from the sinus node and causes a P wave on the surface ECG that is normal in terms of both amplitude and vector. These P waves are typically followed by a normal QRS complex and T wave.

Commonly, sinus bradycardia is an incidental finding in otherwise healthy individuals, particularly in athletes and young adults or sleeping patients. Apart from fit, but otherwise normal, individuals, there is a long list of situations where sinus bradycardia occurs, including:

- Hypothermia
- Increased vagal tone (as a result of vagal stimulation or drugs)
- Hypothyroidism
- β Blockade
- Marked intracranial hypertension
- Obstructive jaundice, and even in uraemia
- Structural SA node disease or ischaemia
- Sleep apnoea
- Hypoglycaemia
- Inferior wall myocardial infarction.

2.33

Answer: D

Primary aldosteronism (Conn's syndrome) is a condition of hyperaldosteronism originating in the adrenal gland. The causes include an aldosterone-secreting adrenocortical adenoma, hyperplasia of the zona glomerulosa and, very rarely, an adrenal carcinoma. It is characterised by hypertension secondary to sodium retention, hypokalaemia and a decreased serum renin caused by a negative feedback of increased blood pressure on renin secretion.

Cushing's syndrome is the result of increased glucocorticoid production, particularly cortisol. Physical signs typically include 'moon facies,' truncal obesity, 'buffalo hump' and purple abdominal striae. Diabetes mellitus is a condition of inadequate insulin production that presents with hyperglycaemia and ketoacidosis. Phaeochromocytoma is a rare tumour of chromaffin cells occurring most commonly in the adrenal medulla. The tumour secretes adrenaline and noradrenaline, resulting in secondary hypertension. Secondary aldosteronism results from an activation of the renin–angiotensin system caused by renal ischaemia, oedema and renal tumours. In contrast to primary aldosteronism, secondary aldosteronism is associated with increased serum renin.

2.34

Answer: E

Renal plasma flow can be determined by the principle of conservation and the use of a substance that is not synthesised or metabolised by the kidney. The amount of such a substance entering the kidney per unit time via the renal artery equals the amount leaving via the ureter and the renal vein. The difficulty of obtaining renal venous plasma samples limits the usefulness of this approach to measuring renal plasma flow. However, it has been found that the tubular secretory system for *p*-aminohippuric acid (PAH) is so efficient that at low plasma concentrations it removes 90% or more of the PAH from the plasma as it flows through the kidney. Thus, for practical reasons, the 10% that remains in the renal vein is ignored and it is assumed that the amount entering the kidneys (renal plasma flow [RPF] x arterial concentration [P_{PAH}]) equals the amount leaving via the ureters:

Urine concentration (U_{PAH}) x Urine flow rate [V, ml/min], ie

$$RPF \times P_{PAH} = U_{PAH} \times V$$

and

$$RPF = U_{PAH} \times V/P_{PAH}$$

So, in this patient, substituting appropriate values, we have (13 mg/ml x 1.0 ml/min)/0.02 mg/ml = 650 ml/min.

2.35

Answer: A

This woman has a risk profile (female, fat, 40s) and symptomatology consistent with gallstones (cholelithiasis). As would be expected, contraction of the gallbladder after a fatty meal often exacerbates the pain caused by gallstones. Cholecystokinin, the release of which is stimulated by dietary fat, is the hormone responsible for stimulation of gallbladder contraction. It is produced in I-cells of the duodenum and jejunum. In addition to gallbladder contraction, cholecystokinin also stimulates pancreatic enzyme secretion and decreases the rate of gastric emptying.

Gastrin is produced by the G-cells of the antrum and duodenum. Gastrin stimulates the secretion of HCl from the parietal cells and pepsinogen from the chief cells of the stomach. Gastrin secretion is stimulated by gastric distension, digestive products (eg amino acids) and vagal discharge. Pepsin is a protease produced by the chief cells of the stomach (as pepsinogen). It is involved in the digestion of proteins. Pepsinogen release is stimulated by vagal stimulation, gastrin, local acid production, secretin, cholecystokinin and histamine. Secretin is produced by the S-cells of the duodenum. It is secreted primarily in response to acidification of the duodenal mucosa. Secretin stimulates the secretion of bicarbonate-containing fluid from the pancreas and biliary ducts. This neutralisation allows pancreatic enzymes to function. Secretin also inhibits gastric acid production and gastric emptying. Somatostatin is produced by the D-cells of the pancreatic islets and in the gastric and intestinal mucosa. Somatostatin is an inhibitory hormone; it inhibits the secretion of most gastrointestinal hormones, gallbladder contraction, gastric acid and pepsinogen secretion, pancreatic and small intestinal fluid secretion and both glucagon and insulin release.

2.36

Answer: B

Adult humans produce 400–800 ml of bile daily. The secretion of bile can be considered to occur in two stages:

1. Initially, hepatocytes secrete bile into canaliculi, from which it flows into bile ducts. This hepatic bile contains large quantities of bile acids, cholesterol and other organic molecules.
2. As bile flows through the bile ducts it is modified by addition of a watery, bicarbonate-rich secretion from ductal epithelial cells.

Bile acids are derivatives of cholesterol synthesised in the hepatocyte. Cholesterol, ingested as part of the diet or derived from hepatic synthesis, is converted into the bile acids cholic and chenodeoxycholic acids, which are then conjugated to an amino acid (glycine or taurine) to yield the conjugated form that is actively secreted into the canaliculi. Bile acids are facial amphipathic, ie they contain both hydrophobic (lipid soluble) and polar (hydrophilic) faces. The cholesterol-derived portion of a bile acid has one face that is hydrophobic (the one with methyl groups) and one that is hydrophilic (the one with the hydroxyl groups); the amino acid conjugate is polar and hydrophilic. Their amphipathic nature enables bile acids to emulsify lipid aggregates. Bile acids have detergent action on particles of dietary fat, which causes fat globules to break down or be emulsified into minute, microscopic droplets. Emulsification is not digestion as such, but is of importance because it greatly increases the surface area of fat, making it available for digestion by lipases, which cannot access the inside of lipid droplets.

Bile acids are also lipid carriers and are able to solubilise many lipids by forming micelles — aggregates of lipids such as fatty acids, cholesterol and monoglycerides — that remain suspended in water. Bile acids are also critical for transport and absorption of the fat-

physiology

soluble vitamins. Large amounts of bile acids are secreted into the intestine every day, but only relatively small quantities are lost from the body. This is because about 95% of the bile acids delivered to the duodenum are absorbed back into the blood within the ileum. Venous blood from the ileum goes straight into the portal vein, and hence through the sinusoids of the liver. Hepatocytes extract bile acids very efficiently from sinusoidal blood and little escapes the healthy liver into the systemic circulation. Bile acids are then transported across the hepatocytes to be re-secreted into the canaliculi. The net effect of this enterohepatic recirculation is that each bile salt molecule is reused about 20 times, often two or three times during a single digestive phase.

2.37

Answer: C

Cholecystokinin plays a key role in facilitating digestion within the small intestine. It is secreted from mucosal epithelial cells in the first segment of the small intestine (duodenum), and stimulates delivery into the small intestine of digestive enzymes from the pancreas and bile from the gallbladder. It is a linear peptide that is synthesised as a pre-prohormone, and then proteolytically cleaved to generate a family of peptides with the same carboxy ends. Partially digested fats and proteins in the lumen of the duodenum release cholecystokinin which:

- Stimulates secretion of pancreatic enzymes
- Stimulates gallbladder contraction
- Relaxes the sphincter of Oddi
- Inhibits gastric emptying
- Stimulates small bowel motility
- Enhances secretin stimulation of pancreatic bicarbonate secretion.

2.38

Answer: D

The clinical presentation is classic for a glucagonoma, which is a rare neuroendocrine tumour with almost exclusive pancreatic localisation. Malignant glucagonomas are islet cell pancreatic tumours that are discovered because of the glucagonoma syndrome or local mass effects, or incidentally. Glucagonomas originate from the α_2 cells of the pancreas. This tumour is characterised by glucagon overproduction, diabetes mellitus, hypoaminoacidaemia, weight loss, normochromic and normocytic anaemia, and a necrolytic migrating erythema, which is the most characteristic clinical sign of this pathology. Physiological glucagon activity includes:

- Activation of gluconeogenesis
- Stimulation of lipolysis
- Stimulation of catecholamine secretion
- Activation of glycogenolysis with contemporary glycolysis inhibition
- Inhibition of the gastric secreting activity
- Inhibition of the pancreatic secreting activity
- Inhibition of the gastrointestinal motility
- Stimulation of urinary excretion of water and phosphates as well as Na^+, Ca^{2+} and Mg^{2+}.

When glucagon production is a result of a secreting tumour, it becomes independent and loses the feedback control mechanisms, and the subsequent increase of glucagon concentration in the blood causes the symptoms. Diabetes mellitus occurs in patients with a glucagonoma because of the lack of equilibrium between insulin production and glucagon production, which occurs when there are high serum levels of glucagon and normal levels of insulin or when insulin production is reduced and a normal glucagon level is present. However, glucagon may not induce hyperglycaemia directly unless metabolism of glucose by the liver is compromised directly.

physiology

2.39

Answer: E

Macronutrients and micronutrients are absorbed along the length of the small intestine. However, as the jejunum has taller villi, deeper crypts and greater enzyme activity compared with the ileum under normal conditions, about 90% of digestion and absorption of significant macronutrients and micronutrients are accomplished in the proximal 100–150 cm of the jejunum. This includes absorption of proteins, carbohydrates, fats, vitamins B and C and folic acid, and the fat-soluble vitamins A, D, E and K.

The ileum is the site for absorption of water and electrolytes. In addition, the terminal ileum is the site of absorption of bile salts and vitamin B_{12}. Water is also absorbed from the colon. Colonic water absorption could be increased to as much as five times its normal capacity after small bowel resection.

2.40

Answer: A

The pathophysiological changes that follow pulmonary embolism (PE) involve derangements in pulmonary haemodynamics, gas exchange and mechanics. The change in cardiopulmonary function is proportional to the extent of obstruction, which varies with the size and number of emboli obstructing the pulmonary arteries, and to the patient's pre-embolic cardiopulmonary status. The resulting physiological changes may include pulmonary hypertension with right ventricular failure and shock, dyspnoea with tachypnoea and hyperventilation, arterial hypoxaemia and pulmonary infarction. Tachypnoea, often with dyspnoea, almost always occurs after a PE. It appears to be a result of stimulation of juxtacapillary receptors in the alveolar capillary membrane by swelling of the alveolar interstitial space. This stimulation increases reflex vagal afferent activity, which stimulates medullary respiratory neurons. Consequent alveolar hyperventilation is manifested by a lowered $Paco_2$. After occlusion of the pulmonary artery, areas of the lung are ventilated but not perfused, resulting in wasted ventilation with an increased ventilation/perfusion ratio – the physiological hallmark of PE

physiology

– contributing further to the hyperventilatory state. Depletion of alveolar surfactant within hours of the embolic event results in diminished lung volume and compliance. Reduced lung volume secondary to atelectasis or infarction after PE may be manifest on the chest radiograph by diaphragmatic elevation. Diminished lung volume and possibly lowered airway $Paco_2$ may induce bronchoconstriction, leading to expiratory wheezing. Arterial hypoxaemia typically occurs with diminished arterial O_2 saturation (Sao_2 from 94% to 85%), although the Sao_2 may be normal. Hypoxaemia is caused by right-to-left shunting in areas of partial or complete atelectasis not affected by embolisation. A ventilation/perfusion imbalance probably also contributes to hypoxaemia. The mechanisms responsible for the ventilation/perfusion imbalance and atelectasis are not fully defined. In massive PE, severe hypoxaemia may result from right atrial hypertension that causes right-to-left shunting of blood through a patent foramen ovale. Low venous O_2 tension may also contribute to development of arterial hypoxaemia.

2.41

Answer: D

The carotid and aortic bodies are able to monitor the physically dissolved O_2 and CO_2 and the H^+ concentration of arterial blood. These chemoreceptors are stimulated by a decline in the Po_2, especially when it falls below 8 kPa (60 mmHg). They are also stimulated by an increase in the arterial blood H^+ concentration (decreased pH) or an increase in physically dissolved CO_2 (or Pco_2). Although it is not clear precisely how increases in H^+ or CO_2 or decreases in the Po_2 stimulate the chemoreceptors, the peripheral chemoreceptors are the only sensors capable of detecting a fall in the Po_2. Thus, the peripheral chemoreceptors account for increases in ventilation resulting from hypoxia. However, these chemoreceptors detect only levels of physically dissolved O_2 and not the O_2 that is chemically attached to haemoglobin. In contrast to the peripheral receptors, the central chemoreceptors are not sensitive to changes in the Po_2 of cerebral blood or CSF.

2.42

Answer: C

The best diagnostic test for evaluating patients with suspected chronic obstructive pulmonary disease (COPD) is lung function measured with spirometry. Key spirometric measures may be obtained with a portable office spirometer and should include forced vital capacity (FVC) and the normal forced expiratory volume in the first second of expiration (FEV_1). The ratio of FEV_1 to forced vital capacity (FEV_1/FVC) normally exceeds 0.75. Patients with COPD typically present with obstructive airflow. A FEV_1/FVC ratio < 70% in a patient with a postbronchodilator FEV_1 < 80% of the predicted value is diagnostic for COPD. Severity is further stratified based on symptoms and FEV_1 values. A patient with severe disease has a FEV_1 < 50% of the predicted value; values below 30% of the predicted value represent very severe disease. Beyond office spirometry, complete pulmonary function testing may show increased total lung capacity (TLC), functional residual capacity (FRC) and residual volume (RV). A substantial loss of lung surface area available for effective oxygen exchange causes diminished carbon monoxide diffusion in the lung (D_{LCO}) in patients with emphysema. This finding may help distinguish COPD from asthma, because patients with asthma typically have normal D_{LCO} values.

2.43

Answer: B

The glomerular filtration rate (GFR) is generally considered the best measure of renal function despite the fact that the kidney performs an array of duties, including salt and water balance, erythropoiesis, bone metabolism, electrolyte homeostasis and blood pressure control. GFR is traditionally measured as the renal clearance of a particular substance from plasma and is expressed as the volume of plasma that can be completely cleared of that substance in a unit of time. The ideal marker for GFR determinations would appear endogenously in the plasma at a constant rate, be freely filtered at the glomerulus, be neither reabsorbed nor secreted by the renal tubule and undergo no extrarenal elimination. GFR is calculated as follows:

U_x = concentration of x in a timed urine collection (mg/ml)

V = volume of urine per unit time (ml/min)

P_x = concentration of x in plasma (mg/ml)

U_xV = rate of urinary excretion of x = excreted load (mg/min)

$C_x = U_xV/P_x$ = the (plasma) clearance of x (ml/min)

C_x is the volume of plasma containing x that would have to be completely cleared of x per unit time to supply an amount of x for urinary excretion at the measured rate. Clearance does not necessarily mean that an actual volume of plasma is, in fact, completely cleared of x. Rather, it refers to a 'virtual volume' of plasma that would provide the measured amount of x.

A substance that is freely filtered and undergoes neither reabsorption nor secretion will have a clearance equal to the GFR. The clearance of inulin, a carbohydrate polymer of fructose, measured during a constant infusion, is the standard for measurement of GFR. A clearance greater than that of inulin indicates that a substance also undergoes tubular secretion; a clearance less than that of inulin implies tubular reabsorption.

Rewriting the clearance equation for x:inulin, we have:

$$C_{inulin}:U_{inulin} \times V/P_{inulin}$$

As a result of the difficulty in performing inulin clearance, the clearance of endogenous creatinine is used for clinical purposes as an estimate of the GFR. Its plasma concentration remains stable during a 24-hour period and its rate of excretion does not vary with urine flow. Thus, creatinine clearance (C_{cr}) can be calculated during a 24-hour collection of urine, with a plasma sample obtained at any time during the collection period. In a normal man, filtered creatinine does not undergo tubular reabsorption; some tubular secretion does occur. At the plasma creatinine concentration that prevails at a normal GFR, the ration C_{cr}/C_{inulin} is close to 1, implying negligible secretion. At progressively lower GFRs, however, tubular secretion plays an increasingly important part in creatinine excretion. At GFRs < 30 ml/min, C_{cr} may overestimate C_{inulin} by 50–80%.

Blood urea is generally recognised to be a poor measure of renal function, in that it possesses few of the attributes of an ideal marker

physiology

of GFR. It is produced at variable rates, is affected by a number of disease states (congestive heart failure, malnutrition, hyperalimentation) and undergoes renal tubular reabsorption. PAH is used for estimation of the renal plasma flow rate. ^{51}Cr-labelled EDTA, has been used as a reliable measure of glomerular filtration but is costly, involves special specimen handling and requires radiation exposure.

2.44

Answer: E

Oliguria is hypotension or hypovolaemia until otherwise proved. This patient is likely to be hypovolaemic as well as vasoplegic secondary to fluid loss in the abdomen and release of inflammatory mediators (particularly inducible nitric oxide synthase) as a result of faecal soiling. The best strategy will be to give her a fluid challenge with 200–250 ml of colloid solution followed by infusion of noradrenaline, which is a vasopressor. Unless the low urinary output is the result of poor cardiac performance, there is little to be learned by insertion of a Swan–Ganz catheter. If there is concern that this patient had a history of coronary arterial disease, and may have had a perioperative myocardial event, a stroke volume monitor may be useful. Inotrope may be indicated if the patient has poor ventricular function. Corticosteroids have no role in this clinical scenario.

2.45

Answer: C

The diagnosis is acute rhabdomyolysis after reperfusion. The ischaemia–reperfusion injury causes swelling and destruction of muscle cells, leading to the release of cellular contents into the circulation. The mechanism of injury appears to be calcium influx, free radical generation, disruption of the microcirculation, and release of cytotoxic materials and proteases into the local environment. The result is acidosis, hyperkalaemia, hyperphosphataemia and a massive increase in circulating myoglobin levels. Usually myoglobin is reabsorbed by the proximal tubule and metabolised, releasing free iron that is soaked up by glutathione, but in rhabdomyolysis this mechanism is overwhelmed. Free iron generates free radicals, which are nephrotoxic. In addition, in the presence of acidic urine, myoglobin binds with a renal excretory protein (Tamm–Horsfall) to form casts that obstruct the tubules and cause acute tubular necrosis. The diagnosis can be made by measuring serum creatine kinase levels and checking urinary myoglobin (the urine is usually tea coloured).

2.46

Answer: A

At this level, the lateral portion of the dorsal columns (dorsal funiculus) is composed of the fasciculus cuneatus. Axons carrying tactile, proprioceptive and vibratory information from the ipsilateral arm enter the spinal cord via the dorsal root, ascend the cord in the fasciculus cuneatus and synapse in the nucleus cuneatus of the caudal medulla. Secondary neurons from this nucleus give rise to internal arcuate fibres, which decussate and ascend to the thalamus (ventral posterolateral nucleus or VPL) as the medial lemniscus. Tertiary neurons from the VPL project to the ipsilateral somatosensory cortex. Therefore, damage to the fasciculus cuneatus would result in a deficit in tactile, proprioceptive and vibratory sensations in the ipsilateral arm, because the fibres that carry this information do not cross until they reach the medulla.

Fine motor control of the fingers is principally carried by the ipsilateral corticospinal tract in the lateral funiculus of the cord. Motor control of the contralateral foot is carried by the ipsilateral corticospinal tract in the lateral funiculus of the cord. Hemianhidrosis (lack of sweating) of the face could be produced by interruption of sympathetic innervation to the face. The hypothalamospinal tract projects from the hypothalamus to the intermediolateral cell column at levels T1–2. It descends the cord in the lateral funiculus. Interruption of this tract results in Horner's syndrome (miosis, ptosis, hemianhidrosis). Proprioception from the ipsilateral leg is carried by fasciculus gracilis in the medial part of the dorsal columns.

physiology

2.47

Answer: C

The development of acute respiratory distress syndrome (ARDS) starts with damage to the alveolar epithelium and vascular endothelium, resulting in increased permeability to plasma and inflammatory cells into the interstitium and alveolar space and in lung oedema. Damage to the surfactant-producing type II cells and the presence of protein-rich fluid in the alveolar space disrupt the production and function of pulmonary surfactant, leading to microatelectasis and impaired gas exchange. The pathophysiological consequences of lung oedema in ARDS include a decrease in lung volumes, compliance and large intrapulmonary shunts (blood perfusing unventilated segments of the lung). A fall in the RV is uniformly present and contributes to ventilation/perfusion inequality. It has been hypothesised that a defective surfactant may be partially responsible for the small lung volumes and that it may worsen oedema accumulation in ARDS (as increases in alveolar surface tension have been shown to increase lung water content by lowering interstitial hydrostatic pressure and increasing interstitital oncotic pressure. The decrease in lung compliance is secondary to the increased lung recoil pressure of the oedematous lung, which clinically increases the work of breathing and leads to respiratory muscle fatigue.

2.48

Answer: D

Parathyroid hormone is the most important endocrine regulator of calcium and phosphorus concentration in extracellular fluid. This hormone is secreted from cells of the parathyroid glands and finds its major target cells in bone and the kidneys. It stimulates osteoclasts to resorb bone mineral, liberating calcium into the blood. It facilitates calcium absorption from the small intestine indirectly by stimulating production of the active form of vitamin D in the kidney. Vitamin D induces synthesis of a calcium-binding protein in intestinal epithelial cells, which facilitates efficient absorption of calcium into the blood. In addition to stimulating fluxes of calcium into the blood from bone and the intestine, parathyroid hormone puts a brake on excretion of

physiology

calcium in the urine, thus conserving calcium in the blood. This effect is mediated by stimulating tubular reabsorption of calcium. Another effect of parathyroid hormone on the kidney is to stimulate loss of phosphate ions in the urine. Parathyroid hormone is released in response to low extracellular concentrations of free calcium. Changes in blood phosphate concentration can be associated with changes in parathyroid hormone secretion, but this appears to be an indirect effect and phosphate itself is not a significant regulator of this hormone. When calcium concentrations fall below the normal range, there is a steep increase in secretion of parathyroid hormone. Low levels of the hormone are secreted even when blood calcium levels are high.

2.49

Answer: E

Hypoxic pulmonary vasoconstriction is a local response to hypoxia, resulting primarily from constriction of small muscular pulmonary arteries in response to reduced alveolar oxygen tension. This unique response of pulmonary arterioles results in a local adjustment of perfusion to ventilation. This means that, if a bronchiole is obstructed, the lack of oxygen causes contraction of the pulmonary vascular smooth muscle in the corresponding area, shunting blood away from the hypoxic region to better-ventilated regions. Skeletal muscle, heart, kidney and gut arteries all dilate under hypoxic conditions, resulting in increased blood flow to these organs.

2.50

Answer: B

Tissue plasminogen activator (tPA) directly catalyses the proteolytic conversion of plasminogen to plasmin. Alteplase (tPA, Activase) was the first recombinant tissue-type plasminogen activator and is identical to native tissue plasminogen activator. In vivo, tissue-type plasminogen activator is synthesised and made available by cells of the vascular endothelium. It is the physiological thrombolytic agent responsible for most of the body's natural efforts to prevent excessive thrombus propagation. Alteplase is the fibrinolytic agent most

physiology

familiar to A&E and is the lytic agent most often used for the treatment of coronary artery thrombosis, pulmonary embolism and acute stroke. In theory, alteplase should be effective only at the surface of fibrin clot. In practice, however, a systemic lytic state is seen, with moderate amounts of circulating fibrin degradation products and a substantial systemic bleeding risk. The agent may be readministered as necessary, because it is not antigenic and almost never associated with any allergic manifestations.

2.51

Answer: E

Bilirubin is a tetrapyrrole created by the normal breakdown of haem. Most bilirubin is produced during the breakdown of haemoglobin and other haemoproteins. Accumulation of bilirubin or its conjugates in body tissues produces jaundice, which is characterised by high plasma bilirubin levels and deposition of yellow bilirubin pigments in the skin, sclerae, mucous membranes and other less visible tissues. As bilirubin is highly insoluble in water, it must be converted into a soluble conjugate before elimination from the body. In the liver, uridine diphosphate (UDP)-glucuronyl transferase converts bilirubin to a mixture of monoglucuronides and diglucuronides, referred to as conjugated (direct) bilirubin, which is then secreted into the bile by an ATP-dependent transporter. This process is highly efficient under normal conditions, so plasma unconjugated bilirubin concentrations remain low. Normal serum values of total bilirubin are typically 0.2–1 mg/dl (3.4–17.1 mmol/l), of which no more than 0.2 mg/dl (3.4 mmol/l) directly reacts. Conjugated hyperbilirubinaemia results from reduced secretion of conjugated bilirubin into the bile, as occurs in patients with hepatitis, or from impaired flow of bile into the intestine, as occurs in patients with biliary obstruction caused by tumours in the head of the pancreas. Bile formation is very sensitive to a variety of hepatic insults, including high levels of inflammatory cytokines as may occur in patients with septic shock. Diseases that increase the rate of bilirubin formation, such as haemolysis, or diseases that reduce the rate of bilirubin conjugation, such as Gilbert's syndrome, produce unconjugated hyperbilirubinaemia.

physiology

2.52

Answer: C

Stroke volume is calculated by using the following formula:

Cardiac output (CO) = Stroke volume (SV) x Heart rate (HR)

Cardiac output is calculated by using the following formula based on Fick's principle:

$$VO_2 = Q\,(Cao_2 - C\bar{v}o_2)$$

where VO_2 is oxygen consumption, Q-cardiac output, Cao_2 = arterial oxygen content and $C\bar{v}o_2$ = mixed venous oxygen content, respectively.

Substituting the values in this formula we get:

300 ml/min = Q x [(20 − 15) ml]/100 ml

Q = [(300 x 100)/5] ml/min

Q = 6000 ml/min

Next, stroke volume is calculated as follows:

6000 ml/min = SV x 100 beats/min

SV = [6000/100] ml/min

SV = 60 ml/min.

physiology

2.53

Answer: A

Under normal resting conditions, about 5% of the cardiac output goes to the heart, 15% to the brain, 20% to the skin and skeletal muscles, 30% to the gastrointestinal tract and 20% to the kidneys. However, when normalised by weight, the kidneys receive the largest specific blood flow (400 ml/min per 100 g) at rest and are particularly at risk during haemorrhagic shock. The brain also receives a relatively high specific blood flow (50 ml/min per 100 g) as does the heart (60 ml/min per 100 g). Blood flow through the skin varies between 1 and 100 ml/min per 100 g and serves temperature regulation. Skeletal muscle under resting conditions has low specific blood flow ranging between 1 and 2 ml/min per 100 g which may increase up to 20-fold during heavy exercise.

2.54

Answer: E

Growth hormone (GH), also known as somatotrophin, is a protein hormone of about 190 amino acids that is synthesised and secreted by cells called somatotrophs in the anterior pituitary. It is a major participant in control of several complex physiological processes, including growth and metabolism. GH is also of considerable interest as a drug used in both humans and animals. It has important effects on protein, lipid and carbohydrate metabolism. In general, GH stimulates protein anabolism in many tissues. This effect reflects increased amino acid uptake, increased protein synthesis and decreased oxidation of proteins. GH enhances the utilisation of fat by stimulating triglyceride breakdown and oxidation in adipocytes. It is one of a battery of hormones that serves to maintain blood glucose within a normal range. GH is often said to have anti-insulin activity, because it suppresses the abilities of insulin to stimulate uptake of glucose in peripheral tissues and enhances glucose synthesis in the liver.

physiology

2.55

Answer: D

Dehydration describes a state of negative fluid balance that may be caused by decreased intake, increased output (renal, gastrointestinal or insensible losses) or fluid shift (ascites, effusions and capillary leak states such as burns and sepsis). The decrease in total body water causes reductions in both the intracellular and extracellular fluid volumes. Clinical manifestations of dehydration are most closely related to intravascular volume depletion. As dehydration progresses, hypovolaemic shock ultimately ensues, resulting in end-organ failure and death. In acute dehydration, plasma osmolality is increased as more water than salt is lost. The decrease in total body water and plasma volume leads to an inhibition of the baroreceptors and a lower firing rate. The increase in plasma osmolality leads to increased ADH secretion and high plasma ADH levels, which increases the water permeability of collecting duct cells. This leads to more absorption of water by the kidneys and low renal water excretion.

2.56

Answer: B

The key player in acid secretion is a H^+/K^+ ATPase or 'proton pump' located in the canalicular membrane. This ATPase is magnesium dependent and not inhibited by ouabain. Parietal cells secrete an essentially isotonic solution of pure hydrochloric acid (HCl) containing 150 mmol/l Cl^- and 150 mmol/l H^+ (pH < 1). Intracellular H^+ of parietal cells is 10^{-4} mol/l (pH = 7.0) and active transport is necessary to transport H^+ against this gradient. This is achieved by H^+/K^+ ATPase in the apical membrane, which exchanges H^+ for K^+.

physiology

2.57

Answer: D

The mean corpuscular volume (MCV) measures the mean or average size of individual RBCs. To obtain the MCV, the haematocrit is divided by the total RBC count. The MCV is an indicator of the size of the RBCs. If the MCV is low, the cells are microcytic or smaller than normal. Microcytic red blood cells are seen in iron deficiency anaemia, lead poisoning and the genetic diseases thalassaemia major and minor. If the MCV is high, the cells are macrocytic, or larger than normal. Macrocytic RBCs are associated with pernicious anaemia and folic acid deficiencies. If the MCV is within the normal range, the cells are referred to as normocytic. A patient who has anaemia from an acute haemorrhage would have a normocytic anaemia.

Mean corpuscular haemoglobin (MCH) measures the amount, or the mass, of haemoglobin present in one RBC. The weight of haemoglobin in an average cell is obtained by dividing the haemoglobin by the total RBC count. The result is reported as picograms.

MCH concentration (MCHC) measures the proportion of each cell taken up by haemoglobin. The results are reported in percentages, reflecting the proportion of haemoglobin in the RBCs. The haemoglobin is divided by the haematocrit and multiplied by 100 to obtain the MCHC.

The MCH and MCHC are used to assess whether RBCs are normochromic, hypochromic or hyperchromic. An MCHC < 32% indicates that the RBCs are deficient in haemoglobin concentration. This situation is most often seen with iron deficiency anaemia.

Normal values for erythrocyte indices are:

- MCV:
  - men: 80–98 fl (femtolitres)
  - women: 96–108 fl
- MCH: 17–31 pg
- MCHC: 32–36%.

Anaemias can be classified using erythrocyte indices in the following way:

- MCV, MCH and MCHC normal – normocytic/normochromic anaemia – most often caused by acute blood loss.
- Decreased MCV, MCH and MCHC – microcytic/hypochromic anaemia – most often caused by iron deficiency.
- Increased MCV, variable MCH and MCHC – macrocytic anaemia – most often caused by vitamin B_{12} deficiency (caused by pernicious anaemia) and folic acid deficiency.

2.58

Answer: D

Phaeochromocytoma is a tumour that arises in the adrenal medulla and secretes catecholamines. The principal urinary metabolic products of adrenaline (epinephrine) and noradrenaline (norepinephrine) are the metanephrines, vanillylmandelic acid (VMA) and homovanillic acid (HVA). Normal individuals excrete only very small amounts of these substances in the urine. Normal values for 24 h are as follows: free adrenaline and noradrenaline < 100 μg (< 582 nmol), total metanephrine < 1.3 mg (< 7.1 μmol), VMA < 10 mg (< 50 μmol) and HVA < 15 mg (< 82.4 μmol). In phaeochromocytoma and neuroblastoma, urinary excretion of adrenaline, noradrenaline and their metabolic products increases intermittently. However, excretion of these compounds may also be elevated in coma, dehydration or extreme stress states, in patients being treated with rauwolfia alkaloids, methyldopa or catecholamines, or after ingestion of foods containing large quantities of vanilla, especially if renal insufficiency is present. All of these compounds may be measured in the same urine specimen.

Urinary dehydroepiandrosterone and pregnanetriol excretion is often increased in congenital adrenal hyperplasia. Free urinary cortisol levels are elevated in Cushing's syndrome. Increased urinary excretion of the serotonin metabolite 5-hydroxyindoleacetic acid is seen in functioning carcinoids.

physiology

2.59

Answer: A

MEN 1 is characterised by tumours of the parathyroid gland, pancreatic islet cells and pituitary gland. The gene causing MEN–1 has recently been identified on chromosome 11 and appears to function as a tumour-suppressor gene. The clinical features of the MEN–1 syndrome depend on the pattern of tumour involvement in the individual patient. Hyperparathyroidism is present in at least 90% of affected patients. Asymptomatic hypercalcaemia is the most common manifestation; about 25% of patients have evidence of nephrolithiasis or nephrocalcinosis. In contrast to sporadic cases of hyperparathyroidism, diffuse hyperplasia or multiple adenomas are found more frequently than solitary adenomas.

MEN 2A is characterised by medullary carcinoma of the thyroid, phaeochromocytoma and hyperparathyroidism. The clinical features of MEN 2A depend on the type of tumour present. Almost all patients with the MEN 2A syndrome have medullary carcinoma of the thyroid. Phaeochromocytoma occurs in about 50% of patients within MEN 2A. Hyperparathyroidism is less common than medullary carcinoma of the thyroid or phaeochromocytoma. About 25% of affected patients within MEN 2A have clinical evidence of hyperparathyroidism (which may be long standing), with hypercalcaemia, nephrolithiasis, nephrocalcinosis or renal failure.

The distinctive feature of MEN 2B syndrome is the presence of mucosal neuromas in most, if not all, affected patients. The neuromas appear as small glistening bumps about the lips, tongue and buccal mucosa. The eyelids, conjunctivae and corneas are also commonly involved. Thickened eyelids and diffusely hypertrophied lips are characteristic. Gastrointestinal abnormalities related to altered motility (constipation, diarrhoea and, occasionally, megacolon) are common and thought to result from diffuse intestinal ganglioneuromatosis. About half the reported cases show the complete syndrome with mucosal neuromas, phaeochromocytomas and medullary carcinoma of the thyroid. Less than 10% have neuromas and phaeochromocytomas alone, whereas the remainder have neuromas and medullary carcinoma of the thyroid without phaeochromocytoma.

physiology

Recent genetic studies have mapped the genetic defects in MEN 2A, MEN 2B, familial medullary carcinoma of the thyroid and Hirschsprung's disease to the pericentromeric region of chromosome 10 and have identified mutations in a specific receptor tyrosine kinase gene, *ret*, suggesting that this dominant oncogene is responsible for the abnormalities associated with these conditions.

2.60

Answer: B

Hypocalcaemia is defined as a decrease in total plasma calcium concentration < 8.8 mg/dl (2.2 mmol/l) in the presence of a normal plasma protein concentration. Hypocalcaemia has a number of causes. These include:

- Hypoparathyroidism
- Vitamin D deficiency
- Renal tubular disease
- Renal failure
- Magnesium depletion
- Acute pancreatitis
- Hypoproteinaemia
- Enhanced bone formation with inadequate Ca^{2+} intake
- Septic shock
- Hyperphosphataemia.

Drugs associated with hypocalcaemia include those generally used to treat hypercalcaemia: anticonvulsants (phenytoin, phenobarbital) and rifampin, which alter vitamin D metabolism; transfusion with blood products treated with citrate as well as radiocontrast agents containing the divalent ion-chelating agent EDTA (ethylenediaminetetraacetate).

Magnesium depletion occurring with intestinal malabsorption or dietary deficiency can cause hypocalcaemia. Relative parathyroid hormone (PTH) deficiency and end-organ resistance to its action occur with magnesium depletion, resulting in plasma concentrations of < 0.5 mmol/l; repletion of magnesium improves PTH levels and renal Ca^{2+} conservation.

Sarcoidosis, vitamin D excess, immobilisation and milk-alkali excess are associated with hypercalcaemia.

physiology

2.61

Answer: C

Magnesium (Mg^{2+}) is the fourth most plentiful cation in the body. A 70-kg adult has roughly 1000 mmol Mg^{2+}. About 50% is sequestered in bone and not readily exchangeable with other compartments. The extracellular fluid (ECF) contains only about 1% of total body Mg^{2+}. The remainder resides in the intracellular compartment. Normal plasma Mg^{2+} concentration ranges from 0.70 to 1.05 mmol/l. The maintenance of plasma Mg^{2+} concentration is largely a function of dietary intake and extremely effective renal and intestinal conservation. Within 7 days of initiation of a Mg^{2+}-deficient diet, renal and faecal Mg^{2+} excretion each fall to about 0.5 mmol/24 h. About 70% of plasma Mg^{2+} is ultrafiltered by the kidney; the remainder is bound to protein. As with Ca^{2+}, protein binding of Mg^{2+} is pH dependent. Plasma Mg^{2+} concentration and either total body Mg^{2+} or intracellular Mg^{2+} content are not closely related. However, severe plasma hypomagnesaemia may reflect diminished body stores of Mg^{2+}. A wide variety of enzymes are Mg^{2+} activated or dependent. Mg^{2+} is required by all enzymatic processes involving ATP and is also required by many of the enzymes involved in nucleic acid metabolism. Mg^{2+} is required for thiamine pyrophosphate cofactor activity and appears to stabilise the structure of macromolecules such as DNA and RNA. Mg^{2+} is also related to calcium and potassium metabolism in an intimate but poorly understood way.

2.62

Answer: D

The parasympathetic nervous system (PNS) is one of two divisions of the autonomic nervous system. Sometimes called the 'rest and digest' system, the parasympathetic system conserves energy because it slows the heart rate, increases intestinal and gland activity, and relaxes sphincter muscles in the gastrointestinal tract. Although an oversimplification, it is said that the PNS acts in a reciprocal manner to the effects of the sympathetic nervous system; in fact, in some tissues innervated by both systems, the effects are synergistic.

The PNS uses only acetylcholine (ACh) as its neurotransmitter. The ACh acts on two types of receptors: the muscarinic and nicotinic cholinergic receptors. Most transmissions occur in two stages: when stimulated, the preganglionic nerve releases ACh at the ganglion, which acts on nicotinic receptors of the postganglionic nerve. The postganglionic nerve then releases ACh to stimulate the muscarinic receptors of the target organ. The effects of parasympathetic stimulation are:

- Pupil: constriction (greater depth of focal field)
- Ciliary muscle: constriction (near focus)
- Lacrimal gland: secretion increased
- Submandibular gland: secretion released and increased
- Parotid gland: secretion increased
- Heart: decreased pulse rate and myocardial responsiveness
- Lung: constriction of air passages
- Gut: increased peristaltic and segmentation motility
- Liver: reduced blood glucose generation (from glycogen breakdown)
- Pancreas: insulin release
- Kidney: no innervation
- Urinary bladder: relaxation of sphincter and contraction of bladder wall musculature
- Penis: erection plus sensory facilitation
- Arterioles in general: no innervation
- Arterioles in voluntary muscular system: no innervation
- Piloerector muscles (raise hair or goosebumps): no innervation
- Sweat glands: no innervation.

2.63

Answer: E

An increased heart rate is associated with a shortened Q–T interval. The Q–T interval begins at the onset of the QRS complex and the end of the T wave. It represents the time between the start of ventricular depolarisation and the end of ventricular repolarisation. It is useful as a measure of the duration of repolarisation. The Q–T interval will vary depending on the heart rate, age and gender. It increases with

physiology

bradycardia and decreases with tachycardia. Men have shorter Q–T intervals (0.39 s) than women (0.41 s). The Q–T interval is influenced by electrolyte balance, drugs and ischaemia.

2.64

Answer: A

P waves are caused by atrial depolarisation. In normal sinus rhythm, the SA node acts as the pacemaker. The electrical impulse from the SA node spreads over the right and left atria to cause atrial depolarisation. The P-wave contour is usually smooth, entirely positive and of uniform size. The atrial flutter waves, known as F waves, are larger than normal P waves and they have a saw-toothed waveform. The P-wave duration is normally < 0.12 s and the amplitude is normally < 0.25 mV. A negative P wave can indicate depolarisation arising from the atrioventricular (AV) node. The P–R interval is the time (in seconds) from the beginning of the P wave (onset of atrial depolarisation) to the beginning of the QRS complex (onset of ventricular depolarisation). The normal P–R interval duration range is from 0.12 s to 0.20 s, measured from the initial deflection of the P wave to the initial deflection of the QRS complex. The P–R interval is longer with high vagal tone. A prolonged P–R interval can correspond to impaired AV node conduction.

2.65

Answer: B

About half of patients have diagnostic changes on their initial ECG. An ECG should be performed on any patient who is older than 45 years and experiencing atypical or new epigastric pain or nausea. In younger patients, an ECG should be considered when suggestive symptoms are present. Younger patients are disproportionately represented in missed cases. An ECG is a rapid, low-risk, relatively low-cost measure. Results indicating high probability of acute myocardial infarction (AMI) are ST-segment elevation > 1 mm in two contiguous leads and new Q waves. Results indicating intermediate probability of AMI are ST-segment depression or T-wave inversion, Q waves and ST T-wave abnormalities that are known to be old. Results

physiology

indicating low probability of AMI are normal findings on an ECG; however, normal or non-specific findings on an ECG do not exclude the possibility of AMI.

Localisation of an AMI, based on the distribution of ECG abnormalities, is as follows:

- Inferior wall: II, III, aVF
- Lateral wall: I, aVL, V4–V6
- Anteroseptal: V1–V3
- Anterolateral: V1–V6
- Right ventricular: RV4, RV5
- Posterior wall: R/S ratio > 1 in V1 and V2; T-wave changes (ie upright) in V1, V8 and V9.

2.66

Answer: E

Potassium (K^+) is a major ion of the body. Almost 98% of K^+ is intracellular, with the concentration gradient maintained by the Na^+/K^+ ATPase pump. The ratio of intracellular to extracellular K^+ is important in determining the cellular membrane potential. Small changes in the extracellular K^+ level can have profound effects on the function of the cardiovascular and neuromuscular systems. The normal K^+ level is 3.5–5.0 mmol/l, and total body K^+ stores are about 50 mmol/kg (3500 mmol in a 70-kg person). Potassium homeostasis is maintained predominantly through the regulation of renal excretion. The most important site of regulation is the collecting duct, where aldosterone receptors are present. Hyperkalaemia is defined as a K^+ level > 5.5 mmol/l. Ranges are as follows:

- 5.5–6.0 mmol/l – mild condition
- 6.1–7.0 mmol/l – moderate condition
- > 7.0 mmol/l – severe condition

Hyperkalaemia results from the following:

- Decreased or impaired K^+ excretion: as observed with acute or chronic renal failure (most common), potassium-sparing diuretics, urinary obstruction, sickle cell disease, Addison's disease and systemic lupus erythematosus (SLE).

physiology

- Additions of K$^+$ into extracellular space: as observed with potassium supplements (eg oral and intravenous potassium, salt substitutes), rhabdomyolysis and haemolysis (eg venepuncture, blood transfusions, burns, tumour lysis).
- Transmembrane shifts (ie shifting potassium from the intracellular to extracellular space): as observed with acidosis and medication effects (eg acute digitalis toxicity, β blockers, suxamethonium).
- Fictitious or pseudohyperkalaemia: as observed with improper blood collection (eg ischaemic blood draw from venepuncture technique), laboratory error, leukocytosis and thrombocytosis.

An ECG is essential and may be instrumental in diagnosing hyperkalaemia in the appropriate clinical setting. ECG changes have a sequential progression of effects, which roughly correlate with the potassium level. ECG findings may be observed as follows: early changes of hyperkalaemia include peaked T waves, shortened Q–T interval and ST segment depression. These changes are followed by bundle-branch blocks causing a widening of the QRS complex, increases in the P–R interval and decreased amplitude of the P wave. These changes reverse with appropriate treatment. Without treatment, the P wave eventually disappears and the QRS morphology widens to resemble a sine wave. Ventricular fibrillation or asystole follows. ECG findings generally correlate with the potassium level, but potentially life-threatening arrhythmias can occur without warning at almost any level of hyperkalaemia.

2.67

Answer: A

Phospholipase C is activated by hormones with receptors that are coupled to a pG protein. It converts phosphatidyl inositol to inositol triphosphate (IP$_3$) and diacylglycerol (DAG) by cleaving the phosphoester bond between carbon–3 of glycerol and inositol-4,5-bisphosphate on phosphatidylinositol diphosphate. IP$_3$ and DAG can act on other proteins in cells to increase the activity of enzymes, eg protein kinase C, or on membrane channels such as calcium in the sarcoplasmic reticulum in smooth muscle. Phospholipase C does not directly stimulate reactions that affect activity of protein kinase A, tyrosine kinase or guanylyl cyclase. Phospholipases A_2 are a large family of enzymes that specifically deacylate fatty acids from the second carbon atom of the triglyceride backbone of phospholipids, producing a free fatty acid and a lysophospholipid.

2.68

Answer: B

Pitting oedema is always associated with the retention of sodium and occurs when more than 3 l of interstitial fluid collects. As sodium is limited to the ECF compartment, an excess in total body sodium results in pitting oedema caused by the greater volume of the interstitial space compared with the vascular compartment. Therefore, to reduce the plasma osmolality and produce pitting oedema, there must be a greater gain in water than in sodium.

2.69

Answer: C

Sodium is the major osmotically active cation in the ECF compartment. Most of the proximal reabsorption of Na^+ occurs by active transport and is transcellular. The transcellular pathway consists of the apical and basolateral membranes. The Na^+/K^+ ATPase pump in all cell membranes is responsible for active Na^+ transport (efflux) and active K^+ transport (influx). This enzyme maintains the low intracellular Na^+ concentration and the high extracellular Na^+ concentration. Active transport consumes 30–50% of the energy derived from metabolism in most cells. Although the influx of sodium from the tubular lumen to the proximal tubular cell is in the direction favoured by the electrochemical potential, this transport is mediated by specific membrane carrier proteins and not by simple diffusion. These membrane proteins couple the active movement of other solutes to the passive movement of Na^+. Examples include Na^+–glucose and Na^+–amino acid symporters and a Na^+ antiporter. In each case the potential energy released by downhill transport of Na^+ is used to power the uphill transport of the other substance. These

physiology

transport systems are referred to as Na^+-coupled, secondary, active transport processes. It is important to remember that reabsorption includes not only Na^+ influx from the tubular lumen but also active transport of Na^+ out of the cell into the bloodstream.

2.70

Answer: E

The normal jugular venous pulse (JVP) reflects phasic pressure changes in the right atrium and consists of three positive waves and two negative troughs. The positive presystolic 'a' wave is produced by right atrial contraction and is the dominant wave in the JVP particularly during inspiration. During atrial relaxation, the venous pulse descends from the summit of the 'a' wave. Depending on the P–R interval, this descent may continue until a plateau ('z' point) is reached just before right ventricular systole. More often the descent is interrupted by a second positive venous or 'c' wave, which is produced by a bulging of the tricuspid valve into the right atrium during right ventricular isovolumic systole and by the impact of the carotid artery adjacent to the jugular vein. Following the summit of the 'c' wave, the JVP contour declines, forming the normal negative systolic wave, the 'x' trough. The 'x' descent is a result of a combination of atrial relaxation, the downward displacement of the tricuspid valve during right ventricular systole and the ejection of blood from both the ventricles. The positive, late systolic 'v' wave in the JVP results from the increase in blood volume in the vena cavae and the right atrium during ventricular systole when the tricuspid valve is closed. After the peak of the 'v' wave is reached, the right atrial pressure decreases because of the diminished bulging of the tricuspid valve into the right atrium and the decline in right ventricular pressure that follow tricuspid valve opening. The latter occurs at the peak of the 'v' wave in the JVP.

Following the summit of the 'v' wave, there is a negative descending limb, referred to as the 'y' descent or diastolic collapse, which is caused by the opening of the tricuspid valve and flow of blood into the right ventricle. The initial 'y' descent corresponds to the right ventricular rapid filling phase. The trough of the 'y' wave occurs in early diastole and is followed by the ascending limb of the 'y' wave,

physiology

which is produced by continued diastolic inflow of blood into the right side of the heart. The velocity of this ascending pressure curve depends on the rate of venous return and the distensibility of the chambers of the right side of the heart. When diastole is long, the descending limb of the 'y' wave is often followed by a small, brief, positive wave, the 'h' wave, which occurs just before the next 'a' wave. At times, there is a plateau phase rather than a distinct 'h' wave. With increasing pulse rate the 'y' trough and the 'y' ascent are followed immediately by the next 'a' wave. Usually, there are three visible major positive waves ('a', 'c', 'v') and two negative troughs ('x', 'y') when the pulse rate is below 90 beats/min and the P–R interval is normal. With faster heart rates there is often fusion of some of the pulse waves and an accurate analysis of the waveform is more difficult.

2.71

Answer: D

The 'a' wave in the JVP is absent when there is no effective atrial contraction, such as in atrial fibrillation. In certain other conditions, the 'a' wave may not be apparent. In sinus tachycardia the 'a' wave may fuse with the preceding 'v' wave, particularly if the P–R interval is prolonged. In some patients with sinus tachycardia, the 'a' wave may occur during the 'v' wave or 'y' descent and may be small or absent. In the presence of first-degree heart block, a discrete 'a' wave with ascending and descending limbs is often completed before the first heart sound and the 'ac' interval is prolonged. Large 'a' waves are of considerable diagnostic value. When giant 'a' waves are present with each beat, the right atrium is contracting against an increased resistance. This may result from obstruction at the tricuspid valve (tricuspid stenosis or atresia, right atrial myxoma or conditions associated with increased resistance to right ventricular filling). A giant 'a' wave is more likely to occur in patients with pulmonary stenosis or pulmonary hypertension in whom both the atrial and the right ventricular septa are intact.

Cannon 'a' waves occur when the right atrium contracts while the tricuspid valve is closed during right ventricular systole. Cannon waves may occur either regularly or irregularly and are most common

physiology

in the presence of arrhythmias. The most important alteration of the normally negative systolic collapse ('x' wave) of the JVP is its obliteration or even replacement by a positive wave. This is usually the result of tricuspid regurgitation. In some patients with moderate tricuspid regurgitation, there is a fairly distinct positive wave during the ventricular systole between the 'c' and 'v' waves. This abnormal systolic waveform is usually referred to as a 'v' or 'cv' wave, although it has also been referred to as an 'r' (regurgitant) or 's' (systolic) wave. Normally the 'v' wave is lower in amplitude than the 'a' wave in the JVP. In patients with an atrial septal defect, however, the higher left atrial pressure is transmitted to the right atrium, and the 'a' and 'v' waves are often equal in the right atrium and the JVP. In patients with constrictive pericarditis and sinus rhythm, the right atrial 'a' and 'v' waves may also be equal, but the venous pressure is increased, which is unusual with isolated atrial septal defect. In patients with constrictive pericarditis who are in atrial fibrillation, the 'cv' wave is prominent and the 'y' descent rapid. A venous pulse characterised by a sharp 'y' trough and a rapid ascent to the baseline is seen in patients with constrictive pericarditis or severe right-sided heart failure.

2.72

Answer: E

Ketoacidosis is most commonly associated with type 1 diabetes mellitus. Diabetic ketoacidosis (DKA) is a state of absolute or relative insulin deficiency aggravated by ensuing hyperglycaemia, dehydration and acidosis-producing derangements in intermediary metabolism. The most common causes are underlying infection, disruption of insulin treatment and new onset of diabetes. DKA is typically characterised by hyperglycaemia > 300 mg/dl, low bicarbonate (< 15 mmol/l) and acidosis (pH < 7.30) with ketonaemia and ketonuria. A patient with untreated type 1 diabetes mellitus has low levels of plasma insulin and C peptide caused by β-cell destruction. The absence of insulin, the primary anabolic hormone, means that tissues such as muscle, fat and liver do not take up glucose.

Counterregulatory hormones, such as glucagon, growth hormone and catecholamines, enhance triglyceride breakdown into free fatty acids and gluconeogenesis, which is the main cause for the elevation in serum glucose in DKA. β Oxidation of these free fatty acids leads to increased formation of ketone bodies. Overall, metabolism in DKA shifts from the normal fed state characterised by carbohydrate metabolism to a fasting state characterised by fat metabolism. Secondary consequences of the primary metabolic derangements in DKA include an ensuing metabolic acidosis as the ketone bodies produced by β oxidation of free fatty acids deplete extracellular and cellular acid buffers. The hyperglycaemia-induced osmotic diuresis depletes sodium, potassium, phosphates and water, as well as ketones and glucose. Commonly, the total body water deficit is 10% and the potassium deficit is 5mmol/kg body weight. The total body potassium deficit may be masked by the acidosis, which sustains an increased serum potassium level. The potassium level can drop precipitously once rehydration and insulin treatment start. Urinary loss of ketoanions with brisk diuresis and intact renal function may also lead to a component of hyperchloraemic metabolic acidosis.

2.73

Answer: C

Endothelin (ET-1), which is synthesised by vascular endothelium, is one of the most powerful vasoconstrictor substances known. Vascular smooth muscle contraction is observed at concentrations as low as 10^{-11} mol. An endothelin precursor (big ET-1 or pro-ET-1; 39 amino acids) is cleaved to ET-1 (21 amino acids) by an endothelin-converting enzyme (ECE) found on the endothelial cell membrane. ET-1 can then bind to ET_A receptors found on adjacent vascular smooth muscle cells, leading to calcium mobilisation and smooth muscle contraction. The ET_A receptor is coupled to a G-protein linked to phospholipase C and the formation of IP_3. There are also ET_B receptors located on the vascular smooth muscle, which also produce contraction. ET-1 release is stimulated by angiotensin II, ADH, thrombin, cytokines, reactive oxygen species and shearing forces acting on the vascular endothelium. ET-1 release is inhibited by prostacyclin and atrial natriuretic peptide as well as by nitric oxide. ET-1 has a number of other actions besides vasoconstriction. ET-1 stimulates aldosterone secretion, produces positive inotropy and chronotropy in the heart, decreases renal blood flow and GFR, and releases atrial

physiology

natriuretic peptide. ET-1 has been implicated in the pathogenesis of hypertension, vasospasm and heart failure.

2.74

Answer: B

The juxtaglomerular apparatus (JGA) is a small endocrine organ associated with individual nephrons within the kidneys. It is composed of:

- the macula densa of the proximal distal tubule of the nephron
- the closely situated afferent arteriole of the same nephron.

Two cell types intervene between macula densa and arteriole in the 'mesangial' region:

1. Granular mesangial cells containing prorenin granules, the precursor of renin; they are modified smooth muscle cells that secrete renin into the afferent arteriole
2. Agranular lacis cells.

Sympathetic nerves lie in close proximity to the granular cells.

The JGA is in an ideal position to monitor the amount and composition of urine in the nephron and blood in the afferent arteriole. Renin secretion may be modified accordingly.

Destruction of the JGA results in a decrease in renin production, which causes a reduction in angiotensin II and aldosterone levels. Hypoaldosteronism leads to an inability to reabsorb sodium in the late distal and early collecting ducts (hyponatraemia), inability to excrete potassium (hyperkalaemia) and inability to excrete H^+ (metabolic acidosis) in exchange for sodium.

physiology

2.75

Answer: C

Central venous pressure decreases with deep inspiration, thereby increasing venous return. This is explained by the negative intrathoracic pressure originated at inspiration, which is transmitted to the great veins of the thorax; moreover, the downward diaphragm movement during this phase helps the pulling of blood towards the heart by increasing the intra-abdominal pressure. At expiration, the mechanisms reverse. The end-diastolic volume and stroke volume of the right heart increase. The increased output of the right heart enters a pulmonary circulation in which capacitance has been increased by the decreased intrathoracic pressure. Therefore, venous return to the left atrium does not increase until expiration, at which time the intrapleural pressure becomes less negative. Cardiac output from the left ventricle increases during expiration.

2.76

Answer: A

Vasoconstrictor agents such as noradrenaline or ephedrine act primarily on small veins to increase peripheral venous pressure. This results in increased venous return, increased preload and therefore increased ventricular end-diastolic volume (EDV). An increase in ventricular EDV results in an increased stroke volume, because the ventricle responds to stretch by developing a greater force of contraction ejecting a greater volume. An increase in EDV leads to a decrease in the end-diastolic reserve volume. The sum of all these effects is increased cardiac workload.

physiology

2.77

Answer: B

γ Motor neurons are located in the anterior grey horn of the spinal cord and motor nuclei of the cranial nerves. These stimulate contraction of intrafusal fibres in muscle spindles to regulate their activity. The γ motor neurons are controlled primarily by the neurons in the descending motor tracts from the brain. Most of these neurons are inhibitory, although some are excitatory. Afferents from the muscle spindles (1a afferents) and the Golgi tendon organs do not synapse with the γ motor neurons.

2.78

Answer: E

The transmembrane voltage changes that take place during an action potential result from changes in the permeability of the membrane to specific ions, the internal and external concentrations of which are maintained in an imbalance by cells. In the axon fibres of nerves, depolarisation results from the inward rush of Na^+, whereas repolarisation and hyperpolarisation arise from an outward movement of K^+. Ca^{2+} ions make up most or all of the depolarising currents at an axon's presynaptic terminus, in muscle cells (including those of the heart) and in some dendrites. The imbalance of ions that makes possible not only action potentials but the resting cell potential arises through the work of the pumps, in particular the Na^+/K^+ exchanger. While the cell is at resting cell potential, the electric forces between the Na^+ and K^+ of the neuron is counterbalanced by the diffusive forces, creating a state of equilibrium.

Changes in membrane permeability and the onset and cessation of ionic currents reflect the opening and closing of voltage-gated ion channels, which provide portals through the membrane for ions. Residing in and spanning the membrane, these proteins sense and respond to changes in transmembrane potential. The depolarisation phase of an action potential is the result of the opening of voltage-gated ion channels, either sodium or calcium channels or a combination of both, depending on the particular membrane. As Na^+ and Ca^{2+} are positively charged, when a voltage-gated Na^+ channel or

Ca^{2+} channel opens, these positively charged ions move into the cell. Voltage-gated Na^+ channels automatically gate shut after about a millisecond. Ca^{2+}-mediated action potentials can be much longer in duration. The repolarisation phase of an action potential is the result of the opening of voltage-gated K^+ channels. There is a decrease in Na^+ permeability (inactivation of the voltage-gated Na^+ channels) and a delayed increase in K^+ permeability during the repolarisation phase of the action potential. Cells normally keep the concentration of K^+ high inside cells. When voltage-gated K^+ channels open, positively charged K^+ move out of the cell, causing the membrane potential to return to a negative inside potential. The Na^+/K^+ pump plays no direct role in the action potential.

2.79

Answer: C

Calcium is the so-called 'trigger' for muscle contraction. Calcium aids in the formation of action potential in the motor end-plate, and is later released from the terminal cisternae of the sarcoplasmic reticulum (not the sarcolemma) into the cytosol of a striated (cardiac and skeletal) muscle cells. Next Ca^{2+} binds to troponin which causes a change in the conformation of the troponin–tropomyosin complex that exposes the myosin-binding sites on the actin filament. The myosin heads then attach to the actin filament and muscle contraction occurs.

2.80

Answer: A

Each of the neurons in the various layers of the retina covers an area in your field of vision. This area in space, where the presence of an appropriate stimulus will modify the activity of this neuron, is called the *receptive field* of this neuron. The receptive field of a single photoreceptor cell, for example, can be said to be limited to the tiny spot of light, within your field of vision, that corresponds to this photoreceptor's precise location on your retina. But, in each succeeding layer of the retina, the receptive fields become increasingly complex, and they become even more complex when it

physiology

comes to the neurons of the visual cortex. An example of this complexity is the receptive fields of bipolar cells, which are circular. But the centre and the surrounding area of each circle work in opposite ways: a ray of light that strikes the centre of the field has the opposite effect from one that strikes the area surrounding it (known as the 'surround'). In fact, there are two types of bipolar cells, distinguished by the way they respond to light on the centres of their receptive fields. They are called on-centre and off-centre cells. If a light stimulus applied to the centre of a bipolar cell's receptive field has an excitatory effect on that cell, causing it to become depolarised, it is an on-centre cell. A ray of light that falls only on the surround will, however, have the opposite effect on such a cell, inhibiting (hyperpolarising) it. The other kind of bipolar cells, off-centre cells, display exactly the reverse behaviour: light on the field's centre has an inhibitory (hyperpolarising) effect, whereas light on the surround has an excitatory (depolarising) effect.

2.81

Answer: D

Presbycusis is defined as sensorineural hearing loss that occurs in people as they age and that may be affected by genetic or acquired factors. Presbycusis begins after age 20 but is usually significant only in those aged over 65. Men are affected more often and more severely than women. Stiffening of the basilar membrane and deterioration of the hair cells, stria vascularis, ganglion cells and cochlear nuclei may play a role in pathogenesis, and presbycusis appears to be related in part to noise exposure. It first affects the highest frequencies (18–20 kHz) and gradually affects the lower frequencies; it usually begins to affect the 4- to 8-kHz range by age 55–65, although variation is considerable. Some persons are severely handicapped by age 60, and some are essentially untouched at age 90. The loss of high-frequency hearing makes discrimination of speech particularly difficult. Thus, many people who have this type of loss have difficulty understanding conversation, particularly when background noise is present, and complain that others mumble.

2.82

Answer: B

A muscle fibre is a single cell of a muscle. Muscle fibres contain many myofibrils, the contractile unit of muscles. Muscle fibres are very long; a single fibre can reach a length of 30 cm. Skeletal muscle fibres can be divided into two basic types: type I (slow-twitch) and type II (fast-twitch) fibres. Type I muscle fibres (slow, oxidative fibres) use primarily cellular respiration and, as a result, have relatively high endurance. To support their high-oxidative metabolism, these muscle fibres typically have lots of mitochondria and myoglobin, and thus appear red or what is typically termed 'dark' meat in poultry. Type I muscle fibres are typically found in high endurance muscles such as postural muscles. They are capable of long, sustained contractions without fatigue, and contain scant glycogen. Their size remains unchanged with exercise but conditioning increases enzymes in aerobic glycolysis. They appear pale even with ATPase staining at an alkaline pH.

Type II muscle fibres use primarily anaerobic metabolism and have relatively low endurance. As a result of their low-oxidative demand, these muscle fibres have low levels of mitochondria and myoglobin, and thus appear white. These muscle fibres are typically used during tasks requiring short bursts of strength, such as sprints or weightlifting. Type II muscle fibres cannot sustain contractions for a significant length of time, and are typically found in the white muscle such as the biceps. They are rich in glycogen. They have more enzymes for anaerobic glycolysis than type I fibres, and they hypertrophy with regular training. They appear dark with ATPase staining at an alkaline pH.

2.83

Answer: A

Upper motor neuron lesions are characterised by weakness, spasticity, hyperreflexia, increased muscle tone, primitive reflexes and Babinski's sign. Primitive reflexes include the grasp, suck and snout reflexes. Damage to the upper motor neurons reduces the considerable inhibitory influence that these tracts have on the lower motor

physiology

neurons. As a result, the excitatory influence of reflexes predominates, causing an increase in muscle tone and hyperreflexia. Lower motor neuron lesions are characterised by weakness, hypotonia, hyporeflexia, atrophy and fasciculations. Fasciculations are fine movements of the muscle under the skin and are indicative of lower motor neuron disease. They are caused by denervation of whole motor units leading to ACh hypersensitivity at the denervated muscle. Atrophy of the affected muscle is usually concurrent with fasciculations. Paraesthesia (abnormal sensations) is not a feature of motor neuron lesions.

2.84

Answer: E

Erythropoietin (EPO) is a glycoprotein hormone that is a growth factor for erythrocyte (RBC) precursors in the bone marrow. It increases the number of RBCs in the blood. In adult humans, EPO is produced primarily by peritubular cells in the kidneys, where its production is stimulated by low oxygen levels in the blood. Some EPO is also produced by the liver, which is the primary source in the fetus. EPO acts by binding to a specific erythropoietin receptor (EPO-R) on the surface of red cell precursors in the bone marrow, stimulating them to transform into mature RBCs. As a result the oxygen level in blood reaching the kidney rises and the amount of EPO produced decreases. Synthetic erythropoietin is available as a therapeutic agent produced by recombinant DNA technology. It is used in treating anaemia resulting from either chronic renal failure or chemotherapy for the treatment of cancer. Its use is also believed to be common as a blood-doping agent in endurance sports such as bicycle racing, triathlon and marathon running.

Shift cells are not normally found in the peripheral blood unless the bone marrow is stimulated by EPO or something in the marrow is pushing cells out, such as a metastatic tumour. These cells have a bluish discoloration (polychromasia) on the Wright–Giemsa stain because they have more RNA than a peripheral blood reticulocyte. Shift cells are basophilic staining RBCs that are even younger than peripheral blood reticulocytes. These cells are considered to be marrow reticulocytes as opposed to peripheral blood reticulocytes.

The reticulocyte count is the best index of erythropoiesis, or how well the bone marrow is responding to an anaemia. The reticulocyte count is increased in an erythropoietin-stimulated bone marrow. The normal myeloid:erythroid ratio is 3:1. An increase in RBCs in response to EPO will decrease the ratio. Decreased serum ferritin indicates a decrease in the marrow iron stores, as in iron deficiency. It does not evaluate effective or ineffective erythropoiesis. The radioactive plasma iron turnover will increase in EPO-stimulated bone marrow as radioactively labelled iron will be removed from plasma and delivered to developing normoblasts in the marrow.

2.85

Answer: C

The blood clotting system or coagulation pathway, similar to the complement system, is a proteolytic cascade. Each enzyme of the pathway is present in the plasma as a zymogen, ie an inactive form, which on activation undergoes proteolytic cleavage to release the active factor from the precursor molecule. The coagulation pathway functions as a series of positive and negative feedback loops that control the activation process. The ultimate goal of the pathway is to produce thrombin, which can then convert soluble fibrinogen into fibrin, forming a clot. The generation of thrombin can be divided into three phases: the intrinsic and extrinsic pathways that provide alternative routes for the generation of factor X, and the final common pathway that results in thrombin formation.

The intrinsic pathway is activated when blood comes into contact with either subendothelial connective tissues or a negatively charged surface that is exposed as a result of tissue damage. Quantitatively, it is the most important of the two pathways, but is slower to cleave fibrin than the extrinsic pathway. The Hageman factor (factor XII), factor XI, prekallikrein and high-molecular-weight kininogen (HMWK) are involved in this pathway of activation. Thus, this pathway provides a further example of the interrelationship of the various enzyme cascade systems in plasma.

The first step is the binding of Hageman factor to a subendothelial surface exposed by an injury. A complex of prekallikrein and HMWK interacts with the exposed surface in close proximity to the bound

physiology

factor XII, which becomes activated. During activation, the single-chain protein of the native Hageman factor is cleaved into two chains (50 and 28 kDa), which remain linked by a disulphide bond. The light chain (28 kDa) contains the active site and the molecule is referred to as activated Hageman factor (factor XIIa). There is evidence that the Hageman factor can autoactivate, so the pathway is self-amplifying once triggered (compare with the alternative pathway of complement). Activated Hageman factor in turn activates prekallikrein. The kallikrein produced can then cleave factor XII and a further amplification mechanism is triggered. The activated factor XII remains in close contact with the activating surface, such that it can activate factor XI, the next step in the intrinsic pathway that, to proceed efficiently, requires calcium.

Also involved at this stage is HMWK, which binds to factor XI and facilitates the activation process. Activated factors XIa, XIIa and kallikrein are all serine proteases, as are many of the enzymes of the complement system. Eventually the intrinsic pathway activates factor X, a process that can also be brought about by the extrinsic pathway. Factor X is the first molecule of the common pathway and is activated by a complex of molecules containing activated factor IX, factor VIII, calcium and phospholipid, which is provided by the platelet surface, where this reaction usually takes place. The precise role of factor VIII in this reaction is not clearly understood. Its presence in the complex is obviously essential, as evidenced by the serious consequences of factor VIII deficiency experienced by people with haemophilia. Factor VIII is modified by thrombin, via a reaction that results in greatly enhanced factor VIII activity and promotes the activation of factor X.

The extrinsic pathway is an alternative route for the activation of the clotting cascade. It provides a very rapid response to tissue injury, generating activated factor X almost instantaneously, compared with the seconds or even minutes required for the intrinsic pathway to activate factor X. The main function of the extrinsic pathway is to augment the activity of the intrinsic pathway.

There are two components unique to the extrinsic pathway: tissue factor or factor III, and factor VII. Tissue factor is present in most human cells bound to the cell membrane. The activation process for tissue factor is not entirely clear. Once activated, it binds rapidly to factor VII, which is then activated to form a complex of tissue factor, activated factor VII, calcium and a phospholipid; this complex then rapidly activates factor X.

The intrinsic and extrinsic systems converge at factor X to a single common pathway, which is ultimately responsible for the production of thrombin (factor IIa). The end-result of the clotting pathway is the production of thrombin for the conversion of fibrinogen to fibrin. Fibrinogen is a dimer soluble in plasma. Exposure of fibrinogen to thrombin results in its rapid proteolysis and the release of fibrinopeptide A. The loss of small peptide A is not sufficient to render the resulting fibrin molecule insoluble, a process that is needed for clot formation, but it tends to form complexes with adjacent fibrin and fibrinogen molecules. A second peptide, fibrinopeptide B, is cleaved by thrombin, and the fibrin monomers formed by this second proteolytic cleavage polymerise spontaneously to form an insoluble gel. The polymerised fibrin, held together by non-covalent and electrostatic forces, is stabilised by the transamidating enzyme factor XIIIa, produced by the action of thrombin on factor XIII. These insoluble fibrin aggregates (clots), together with aggregated platelets (thrombi), block the damaged blood vessel and prevent further bleeding.

The coagulation pathway and other plasma enzyme systems are interrelated. Contact activation of the coagulation pathway, in addition to promoting blood clotting, results in the generation of plasminogen activator activity, which is involved in fibrinolysis or clot removal. Activated Hageman factor and its peptides can also initiate the formation of kallikrein from plasma prekallikrein, and this triggers the release of bradykinin from kininogens in the plasma. Kinins are responsible for dilating small blood vessels, inducing a fall in blood pressure, triggering smooth muscle contraction and increasing the permeability of vessel walls. In addition, activation of the coagulation pathway produces a vascular permeability factor, as well as chemotactic peptides for professional phagocytes.

physiology

2.86

Answer: D

Disorders of the cerebellum and its inflow or outflow pathways produce deficits in the rate, range and force of movement. Anatomically, the cerebellum has three subdivisions. The archicerebellum (vestibulocerebellum), comprising the flocculonodular lobe, helps maintain equilibrium and coordinate eye–head–neck movements, and is closely interconnected with the vestibular nuclei. The midline vermis (paleocerebellum) helps coordinate movement of the trunk and legs; vermis lesions result in abnormalities of stance and gait. The lateral hemispheres, which make up the neocerebellum, control ballistic and finely coordinated limb movements, predominantly of the arms. Signs of cerebellar disease include:

- Ataxia: reeling, wide-based gait.
- Decomposition of movement: inability properly to sequence fine, coordinated acts.
- Dysarthria: inability to articulate words properly, with slurring and inappropriate phrasing.
- Dysdiadochokinesia: inability to perform rapid, alternating movements.
- Dysmetria: inability to control range of movement.
- Hypotonia: decreased muscle tone.
- Nystagmus: involuntary rapid oscillation of the eyeballs in a horizontal, vertical or rotary direction with the fast component maximal towards the side of the cerebellar lesion.
- Scanning speech: slow enunciation with a tendency to hesitate at the beginning of a word or syllable.
- Tremor: rhythmic, alternating, oscillatory movements of a limb as it approaches a target (intention tremor) or of proximal musculature when fixed posture or weight bearing is attempted (sustention tremor).

Chorea is brief, purposeless involuntary movements of the distal extremities and face, which may merge imperceptibly into purposeful or semi-purposeful acts that mask the involuntary motion. Athetosis is writhing movements, often with alternating postures of the proximal limbs that blend continuously into a flowing stream of

physiology

movement. Chorea and athetosis often occur together (choreoathetosis). The most important cause of chorea is Huntington's disease. Other causes include thyrotoxicosis, SLE affecting the central nervous system (CNS) and drugs (eg antipsychotics). Chorea and athetosis are manifestations of dopaminergic overactivity in the basal ganglia – the antithesis of Parkinson's disease. Resting tremor is a feature of parkinsonism. Tics are brief, rapid, simple or complex involuntary movements that are stereotypical and repetitive, but not rhythmic. Simple tics (eg blinking) often begin as nervous mannerisms in childhood or later and disappear spontaneously. Complex tics often resemble fragments of normal behaviour.

2.87

Answer: B

Almost 50% of cases of extrahepatic biliary obstruction have a non-calculous cause, with malignancy being the most frequent. Most tumours originate in the head of the pancreas, through which the distal common duct normally courses. Less common tumours may originate in the ampulla, bile duct, gallbladder or liver. Even less commonly, ducts may be obstructed by metastatic tumours or nodes of lymphoma. Benign tumours, usually papillomas or villous adenomas, also occur in bile ducts and may cause obstruction. Obstruction of intrahepatic or extrahepatic bile ducts prevents the normal delivery of conjugated bilirubin to the duodenum. Hence, conjugated bilirubin (direct bilirubin) regurgitates into the blood, producing jaundice.

Conjugated bilirubin is more water soluble than free bilirubin, and can be filtered by the kidney and excreted in the urine. Intestinal bilirubin is usually metabolised by bacteria in the distal small intestine to produce urobilinogen, a portion of which is reabsorbed into the enterohepatic circulation and can be excreted in the urine. Most of the urobilinogen is further metabolised by colonic bacteria to produce stercobilin, which gives the stool its brown colour. In cases of biliary tree obstruction, bilirubin secretion into the duodenum is reduced and, hence, urinary excretion of urobilinogen is decreased and the presence of urobilinogen and stercobilin in the colon is reduced (clay-coloured stools).

physiology

2.88

Answer: E

The endocrine portion of the pancreas takes the form of many small clusters of cells called islets of Langerhans or, more simply, islets. Humans have roughly a million islets. Pancreatic islets house three major cell types, each of which produces a different endocrine product:

- α cells (A cells) secrete the hormone glucagon
- β cells (B cells) produce insulin and are the most abundant of the islet cells
- δ cells (D cells) secrete the hormone somatostatin, which is also produced by a number of other endocrine cells in the body.

Amino acids (especially arginine) stimulate the secretion of both insulin and glucagon. Hypoglycaemia stimulates insulin secretion, but inhibits glucagon release. Glucagon increases hepatic gluconeogenesis and glycogenolysis, whereas insulin inhibits gluconeogenesis and stimulates glycogen synthesis. The activity of hormone-sensitive lipase is increased by glucagon and decreased by insulin.

2.89

Answer: A

Specific gravity measures the kidney's ability to concentrate or dilute urine in relation to plasma. As urine is a solution of minerals, salts and compounds in water, the specific gravity is > 1.000. The more concentrated the urine, the higher the urine specific gravity. An adult's kidneys have a remarkable ability to concentrate or dilute urine. In infants, the range for specific gravity is less because immature kidneys are not able to concentrate urine as effectively as mature kidneys. The conditions associated with increased or decreased urine specific gravity include:

physiology

Increased

- Dehydration
- Fever
- Vomiting
- Diarrhoea
- Diabetes mellitus and other causes of glycosuria
- Congestive heart failure
- SIADH
- Adrenal insufficiency
- X-ray contrast.

Decreased

- Diabetes insipidus
- Excessive hydration
- Glomerulonephritis
- Pyelonephritis
- Diuretics
- Aldosteronism
- Renal insufficiency
- Falsely decreased specific gravity
- Alkaline urine
- Falsely increased specific gravity
- Intravenous dextran or radiopaque dye
- Proteinuria.

A fixed urine specific gravity (isosthenuria) means that it remains the same at all times, usually around 1.010. Fixed specific gravity indicates that the kidneys have no concentration or dilution capability and that the glomerular filtrate is iso-osmotic with the plasma all the way through the nephron. As concentration and dilution are functions of the renal tubules, a fixed specific gravity always indicates major tubular dysfunction, which commonly occurs in chronic renal failure. Isosthenuria has nothing to do with a reduction in solute load, which would decrease the urine volume. Acute glomerulonephritis and prerenal azotaemia both have intact tubular function and normal concentration and dilution capabilities.

physiology

233

2.90

Answer: D

Cardiac arrest may occur at any time during treatment of hyperkalaemia. Hospitalisation and close monitoring are required. The goal of acute treatment is to protect the body from the effects of hyperkalaemia. This may include protective measures, shift of potassium into the ICF and reduction of total body potassium. Emergency treatment is indicated if the potassium is very high or if severe symptoms are present, including changes in the ECG. Intravenous calcium chloride may be given temporarily to counteract the muscular and cardiac effects of hyperkalaemia, including cardiac arrhythmias. Intravenous calcium will counteract symptoms for only about 1 hour, so other treatments should begin immediately. Intravenous glucose and insulin move potassium from the ECF back into the cells. This may reverse severe symptoms long enough to allow correction of the cause of the hyperkalaemia. Sodium bicarbonate causes potassium to shift from ECF to ICF. It may reverse hyperkalaemia caused by acidosis with no other treatment required. Prolonged use of sodium bicarbonate should be avoided because it may cause severe complications.

Diuretics cause a decrease in total body potassium. They may be prescribed for people who can tolerate the loss of body fluid that accompanies use of a diuretic. Cation-exchange resins, such as sodium polystyrene sulphonate, are chemicals that bind potassium and cause it to be excreted from the gastrointestinal tract. They may be given orally or rectally. Haemodialysis may be used to reduce total body potassium levels, especially if kidney function is compromised. Dialysis is indicated when more conservative measures have failed or are inappropriate. Enalapril is an angiotensin-converting enzyme (ACE) inhibitor. It inhibits ACE and the formation of angiotensin II, which reduces aldosterone and thereby increases serum potassium. It is contraindicated in patients with hyperkalaemia.

2.91

Answer: C

Pleural fluid is continuously produced and reabsorbed, essentially maintaining equilibrium. Pleural fluid moves into the pleural space as a result of oncotic and hydrostatic pressure of the systemic circulation. Although the reabsorption rate ranges from 20 to 1000 ml/24 h, at any given time there is only 10 ml fluid in the pleural space. The lymphatic system, particularly that of the parietal pleura, plays an important role in the reabsorption of excess fluid and proteins. The pH is > 7. The protein content is 10–20 g/l with 60% albumin. The pleural fluid lactate dehydrogenase (LDH) is < 50% plasma LDH. The pleural fluid glucose content is the same as the plasma glucose content. The cellular composition of normal pleural fluid is as follows:

- Mesothelial cells: 10–70%
- Monocytes: 30–70%
- Lymphocytes: 5–30%
- Granulocytes: 10%.

2.92

Answer: E

CSF leak may occur from the nose (rhinorrhoea), the external auditory canal (otorrhoea) or a traumatic or surgical defect in the skull or spine. The fluid leak is a result of meningeal dural and arachnoid laceration with fistula formation. Blunt trauma is the most common cause. Normal adult subarachnoid fluid has a circulating volume of 90–150 ml. About 500 ml CSF is produced daily, primarily from the ventricular choroid plexus. Circulating CSF is absorbed into the venous circulation, mainly through the cranial arachnoid granulations and spinal arachnoid villi. Normal CSF pressure is 100–200 mmH$_2$O. The normal CSF protein content is 20–45 mg/dl and the normal CSF glucose range 50–100 mg/dl, which is 60% of the measured serum glucose value. However, nasal mucous secretions and tears also have detectable glucose content. Therefore, tests used to identify CSF by its glucose content are often false positive (in 45–75% of cases). The absence of glucose tends to exclude CSF as the leaking fluid. The enzyme β_2-transferrin is present in CSF and perilymph but not in sinonasal mucus secretions and tears. This feature is the basis for a specific test for CSF based on immunoelectrophoresis.

physiology

2.93

Answer: B

The vestibular system is the system of balance. It is also involved in the function of maintaining visual fixation during head movement and in maintaining posture and lower muscular control. It is made of five sensory organs on each side of the head embedded in the petrous portion of the temporal bone: the superior, posterior and lateral semicircular canals, as well as the utricle and saccule. The semicircular canals are orthogonal to each other, ie at right angles. This is similar to the corner of a box where the three sides meet. The semicircular canals are shaped like a torus. There is a dilated end of each semicircular canal called the ampulla where the sensory organ is located. The lateral canal is inclined from the horizontal plane about 30°. The superior and posterior canals are at roughly 45° angles to the sagittal plane.

Semicircular canals are sensitive to angular accelerations (head rotations). Each semicircular canal is maximally sensitive to motion in the plane of that canal. The canals also act in functional pairs with both canals lying in the same plane. Rotation in that plane will be excitatory to one canal and inhibitory to the other. The left and right lateral canals are one pair. The superior canal on one side is paired with the posterior canal on the opposite side. The otolith organs include the utricle and the saccule. The utricle senses motion in the horizontal plane (eg forward–backward movement, left–right movement, combination thereof). The saccule senses motion in the sagittal plane (eg up–down movement). It lies in the spherical recess on the medial wall of the vestibule and is oriented in the vertical plane. The utricle lies in the elliptical recess on the medial wall of the vestibule and is oriented in the horizontal plane. There are five openings into the area of the utricle from the semicircular canals. The superior and posterior canals share a common crus.

The membranous labyrinth is enclosed in a bony labyrinth within the petrous portion of the temporal bone. It is surrounded by perilymph and contains endolymph. Perilymph may be formed from an utrafiltrate of blood or CSF. It is similar in ionic concentration to ECF with low K^+ and high Na^+. The endolymph within the membranous labyrinth is produced by the marginal cells of the stria vascularis in the cochlea and by cells called dark cells in the maculae of the utricle and saccule. Endolymph is absorbed in the endolymphatic sac. It has ionic concentrations similar to intracellular fluid (ICF) with high K^+ and low Na^+.

The sensory portion of the semicircular canals is the ampulla, which contains the neuroepithelium called the crista ampullaris, the cupula, supporting cells, connective tissue, blood vessels and nerve fibres. The crista extends perpendicularly across the canal in a saddle shape. The sensory hair cells and supporting cells are modified columnar epithelial cells with microvilli. There are two types of hair cells: type I are flask shaped and have a chalice-shaped nerve ending on them. One calyx nerve ending can synapse with just one or two to four hair cells. Type II hair cells are cylindrical in shape and have multiple efferent and afferent bouton nerve synapses. These hair cells have 50–100 stereocilia and a single kinocilium. These stereocilia are not true cilia but microvilli that are graded in height, with the tallest nearest to the single kinocilium. The kinocilium is located on one end of the cell, giving it a morphological polarisation. The movement of the hair bundle towards the kinocilium causes an increase in the firing rate of the hair cell, whereas deflection away causes a decrease in the firing rate. In the lateral semicircular canals the kinocilium is located on the side nearest the utricle whereas in the superior and posterior semicircular canals it is away from the utricle.

The structure of the utricle and saccule differs from the semicircular canals. The sensory portion of the otolith organs is the macula. The cilia from the hair cells extend up to reach the statoconial membrane. This is a gelatinous layer with calcareous particles called otoconia embedded in it. The statoconial membrane has a specific gravity higher than the endolymph and moves with linear acceleration, causing movement of the hair bundles. In the central portion of each statoconial membrane is a line called the striola. In the saccule the hair cells are oriented towards the striola whereas in the utricle they are oriented away from the striola.

physiology

2.94

Answer: A

The anterolateral pathway (also known as the spinothalamic tract) contains two pathways: the anterior spinothalamic tract (neospinothalamic) and the lateral spinothalamic tract (paleospinothalamic). It receives inputs from nociceptors, mechanoreceptors and thermoreceptors. The first-order fibres enter the spinal cord via the dorsal root ganglion; on entering they may travel over a few segments of the spinal cord, forming Lissauer's tract. The first-order fibres synapse with the second-order fibres in the dorsal horn. The second-order fibres decussate in the spinal cord and then ascend in the contralateral anterior or lateral spinothalamic tract. These tracts ascend separately until the medulla, where they run together as the spinal lemniscus. This runs through the pons and midbrain, and synapses with a third-order neuron in the ventral posterolateral nucleus of the thalamus. The third-order neurons leave the thalamus and project to the somatosensory cortex on the postcentral gyrus via the posterior limb of the internal capsule.

The anterior spinothalamic tract mainly mediates sensations of crude touch and the lateral spinothalamic tract mediates sensations of temperature and pain. A lesion of the anterior spinothalamic tract results in contralateral loss of crude touch and pressure sensation below the level of the lesion. A lesion of the lateral spinothalamic tract results in contralateral loss of pain and temperature sensation below the level of the lesion. A lesion of the medial lemniscus pathway results in loss of ability to perceive consciously the position and movements of the ipsilateral limb below the level of damage. There is also impaired muscle control, loss of vibration sensation and loss of discriminatory touch below the level of the lesion.

2.95

Answer: D

Blood enters the liver through two sources: the portal vein and the hepatic artery. The hepatic artery is not an end-artery and has anastomotic channels with the portal vein at several levels of the interlobular regions. The portal area can hold about a quarter of the total blood volume. The average minute flow is 100 ml/100 g liver

physiology

tissue. The hepatic artery supplies about a third to a quarter of the total blood flow and 40% of the oxygen requirement. The portal vein supplies two-thirds to three-quarters of the total blood flow, 60% of oxygen requirement and the major part of nutrition. Pressure in the portal vein is about 8–10 mmHg. Muscular exercise decreases splanchnic blood flow by redistributing blood to the active muscles and brain.

2.96

Answer: E

Broca's area is the section of the human brain (in the opercular and triangular sections of the inferior frontal gyrus of the frontal lobe of the cortex) that is involved in language processing, speech production and comprehension. It can also be described as Brodmann's area 44 (and 45) and is connected to Wernicke's area by a neural pathway called the arcuate fasciculus. Broca's area is named after Pierre Paul Broca, who first described it in 1861, after conducting a post-mortem examination on a speech-impaired patient. There are two main parts of Broca's area, which express different roles during language comprehension and production:

1. Pars triangularis (anterior), which is thought to support the interpretation of various 'modes' of stimuli (plurimodal association) and the programming of verbal conducts.
2. Pars opercularis (posterior), which is thought to support the management of only one kind of stimulus (unimodal association) and the coordination of the speech organs for the actual production of language, given its favourable position close to motor-related areas.

People who have damage to this area may show a condition called Broca's aphasia (sometimes known as expressive aphasia, motor aphasia or non-fluent aphasia), which makes them unable to create grammatically complex sentences: their speech is often described as telegraphic and contains little but content words. Comprehension in Broca's aphasia is relatively normal, although many studies have demonstrated that those with Broca's aphasia have trouble understanding certain kinds of syntactically complex sentences.

physiology

This type of aphasia can be contrasted with Wernicke's aphasia (also known as receptive aphasia) which is characterised by damage to more posterior regions of the left hemisphere (in the superior temporal lobe). Wernicke's aphasia manifests as a more pronounced impairment in comprehension and speech that seems normal grammatically but is often roundabout, vague or meaningless. Global aphasia is characterised by the complete loss of the ability to comprehend spoken or written language, as well as to express language verbally or orthographically. Verbal expression is limited to words or short automatic phrases such as explicatives. Meaning can sometimes appear to be present because of the emotional content of the explicatives, and comprehension is totally absent even though facial expression and fleeting looks might appear that the patient is comprehending. Repetition and naming are also disturbed.

The lesion that typically causes a global aphasia involves the whole perisylvian region in the dominant hemisphere. Usually the damage correlates with an infarction involving the middle cerebral artery. If the cortex is involved, the damage stretches from anterior to Broca's area, deep to the insula, and posterior to the auditory areas and surrounding perisylvian regions. However, the underlying white matter is often also involved. There is usually hemiplegia on the contralateral side, but paresis is not always present. When there is no paresis, recovery tends to be better. Patients with anomic aphasia present with intact repetition, fluent speech and an inability to name things. It may be secondary to recovery from another type of aphasia. Anomic aphasia may represent a mild form of transcortical sensory aphasia, in which other features of semantics are intact. It may be caused by lesions in many brain areas, including the dorsolateral frontal cortex, posterior temporo-occipital cortex and thalamus. A left anterior temporal lesion can also cause anomic aphasia.

2.97

Answer: C

The patient in this question has the classic features of Parkinson's disease (shaking palsy). It is an idiopathic, slowly progressive, degenerative CNS disorder characterised by slow and decreased movement, muscular rigidity, resting tremor and postural instability.

In primary Parkinson's disease, the pigmented neurons of the substantia nigra, locus ceruleus and other brainstem dopaminergic cell groups are lost. The cause is not known. The loss of substantia nigra neurons, which project to the caudate nucleus and putamen, results in depletion of the neurotransmitter dopamine in these areas. Onset is generally after age 40, with increasing incidence in older age groups.

Secondary parkinsonism results from loss of or interference with the action of dopamine in the basal ganglia as a result of other idiopathic degenerative diseases, drugs or exogenous toxins. The most common cause of secondary parkinsonism is ingestion of antipsychotic drugs or reserpine, which produces parkinsonism by blocking dopamine receptors. In 50–80% of patients, the disease begins insidiously with a resting 4- to 8-Hz pill-rolling tremor of one hand. The tremor is maximal at rest, diminishes during movement and is absent during sleep; it is enhanced by emotional tension or fatigue. Usually, the hands, arms and legs are most affected, in that order. Jaw, tongue, forehead and eyelids may also be affected, but the voice escapes the tremor.

In many patients, only rigidity occurs; tremor is absent. Rigidity progresses, and movement becomes slow (bradykinesia), decreased (hypokinesia) and difficult to initiate (akinesia). Rigidity and hypokinesia may contribute to muscular aches and sensations of fatigue. The face becomes mask-like, with the mouth open and diminished blinking, which may be confused with depression. The posture becomes stooped. Patients find it difficult to start walking; the gait becomes shuffling with short steps, and the arms are held flexed to the waist and do not swing with the stride. Steps may inadvertently quicken, and the patient may break into a run to keep from falling (festination). The tendency to fall forwards (propulsion) or backwards (retropulsion) when the centre of gravity is displaced results from loss of postural reflexes. Speech becomes hypophonic, with a characteristic monotonous, stuttering dysarthria. Hypokinesia and impaired control of distal musculature results in micrographia and increasing difficulty with activities of daily living. Dementia affects about 50% of patients, and depression is common.

During examination, passive movement of the limbs is met with a plastic, unvarying, lead-pipe rigidity; superimposed tremor bursts

physiology

may have a ratchet-like cog-wheel quality. The sensory examination is usually normal. Signs of autonomic nervous system dysfunction (eg seborrhoea, constipation, urinary hesitancy, orthostatic hypotension) may be found. Muscle strength is usually normal, although useful power may be diminished and the ability to perform rapid successive movements is impaired. Reflexes remain normal but may be difficult to elicit in the presence of marked tremor or rigidity.

2.98

Answer: D

Testosterone is a steroid hormone from the androgen group. Testosterone is secreted in the testes of men and the ovaries of women. It is the principal male sex hormone and the 'original' anabolic steroid. The effects of testosterone in humans and other vertebrates occur by way of two main mechanisms: by activation of the androgen receptor (directly or as DHT), and by conversion to oestradiol and activation of certain oestrogen receptors. Free testosterone is transported into the cytoplasm of target tissue cells, where it can bind to the androgen receptor, or can be reduced to 5β-dihydrotestosterone (DHT) by the cytoplasmic enzyme 5β-reductase. DHT binds to the same androgen receptor even more strongly than testosterone, so that its androgenic potency is about 2.5 times that of testosterone. The testosterone–receptor or DHT–receptor complex undergoes a structural change that allows it to move into the cell nucleus and bind directly to specific nucleotide sequences of the chromosomal DNA. The areas of binding are called hormone response elements and influence transcriptional activity of certain genes, producing the androgen effects.

The bones and the brain are two important tissues in humans where the primary effect of testosterone is by way of aromatisation to oestradiol. In general, androgens promote protein synthesis and growth of those tissues with androgen receptors. Testosterone effects can be classified as virilising and anabolic effects, although the distinction is somewhat artificial, because many of the effects can be considered both. Anabolic effects include growth of muscle mass and strength, increased bone density and strength, and stimulation of height growth and bone maturation. Virilising effects

physiology

include maturation of the sex organs, particularly the penis and the formation of the scrotum in fetuses, and after birth (usually at puberty) a deepening of the voice, and growth of the beard and torso hair. Many of these fall into the category of male secondary sex characters. Increased testosterone causes deepening of the voice in both sexes at puberty. Testosterone is also often used by bodybuilders and weightlifters to enhance muscle build.

2.99

Answer: A

According to differences in their heavy chain constant domains, immunoglobulins are grouped into five classes, or isotypes: IgG, IgA, IgM, IgD and IgE. IgG is a monomeric immunoglobulin, built of two heavy chains γ and two light chains. Each molecule has two antigen-binding sites. This is the most abundant immunoglobulin and is approximately equally distributed in blood and in tissue liquids. This is the only isotype that can pass through the placenta, thereby providing protection to the fetus in its first weeks of life before its own immune system has developed. It can bind to many kinds of pathogens, eg viruses, bacteria and fungi, and protects the body against them by complement activation (classic pathway), opsonisation for phagocytosis and neutralisation of their toxins. There are four subclasses: IgG1 (66%), IgG2 (23%), IgG3 (7%) and IgG4 (4%). IgG1, IgG3 and IgG4 cross the placenta easily. IgG3 is the most effective complement activator, followed by IgG1 and then IgG2. IgG4 does not activate complement. IgG1 and IgG3 bind with high affinity to Fc receptors on phagocytic cells. IgG4 has intermediate affinity and IgG2 affinity is extremely low.

IgA represents about 15–20% of immunoglobulins in the blood, although it is primarily secreted across the mucosal tract into the stomach and intestines. It is also found in maternal milk, tears and saliva. This immunoglobulin helps to fight against pathogens that contact the body surface and are ingested or inhaled. It does not activate complement and opsonises only weakly. Its heavy chains are of the type α. It exists in two forms – IgA1 (90%) and IgA2 (10%) – that differ in structure.

physiology

IgM forms polymers where multiple immunoglobulins are covalently linked together with disulphide bonds, normally as a pentamer or occasionally as a hexamer. It has a large molecular mass of about 900 kDa (in its pentamer form). The J chain is attached to most pentamers, whereas hexamers do not possess the J chain as a result of space constraints in the complex. As each monomer has two antigen binding sites, an IgM has ten of them; however, it cannot bind ten antigens at the same time because they hinder each other. As it is a large molecule, it cannot diffuse well and is found in the interstitium only in very low quantities. IgM is primarily found in serum; however, because of the J chain, it is also important as a secretory immunoglobulin. As a result of its polymeric nature, IgM possesses high avidity, and is particularly effective at complement activation. It is also a so-called 'natural antibody': it is found in the serum with no evidence of prior contact with antigen.

IgD makes up about 1% of proteins in the plasma membranes of mature naive B lymphocytes (co-expressed with IgM) and is also found in serum in very small amounts. It is monomeric and incorporates the δ heavy chain in its structure. IgD's function is currently unknown, because mice lacking IgD seem to retain normal immune responses (implying redundancy if not lack of function), and IgD ceases to be expressed in activated B lymphocytes. It may function as a regulatory antigen receptor.

IgE is a monomeric immunoglobulin with the heavy chain ε. It contains a high proportion of carbohydrates. Its molecular mass is 190 kDa. It can be found on the surface of the plasma membranes of basophils and mast cells of connective tissue. IgE plays a role in immediate hypersensitivity and the defence against parasites such as worms. The IgE antibodies are also present in outer excretions. They do not activate complement. Only IgE is heat labile.

2.100

Answer: B

The normal blood lactate concentration in unstressed patients is 0.5–1 mmol/l. Patients with critical illness can be considered to have normal lactate concentrations < 2 mmol/l. Hyperlactataemia is defined as a mild-to-moderate (2–5 mmol/l) persistent increase in blood lactate concentration without metabolic acidosis, whereas lactic acidosis is characterised by persistently increased blood lactate levels (usually > 5 mmol/l) in association with metabolic acidosis. Hyperlactataemia generally occurs in the settings of adequate tissue perfusion, intact buffering systems and adequate tissue oxygenation. Lactic acidosis is associated with major metabolic dysregulation, tissue hypoperfusion, effects of certain drugs or toxins or congenital abnormalities in carbohydrate metabolism. Lactic acidosis is divided into two categories: type A and type B (Cohen and Woods). Type A is lactic acidosis occurring in association with clinical evidence of poor tissue perfusion or oxygenation of blood (eg hypotension, cyanosis, cool and clammy extremities). Type B is lactic acidosis occurring when no clinical evidence of poor tissue perfusion or oxygenation exists. The metabolism of glucose to lactate by one tissue, such as RBCs, and conversion of lactate to glucose by another tissue, such as the liver, is termed the 'Cori cycle'. The ability of the liver to consume lactate is concentration dependent and progressively decreases as the level of blood lactate increases.

Lactate uptake by the liver is also impaired by several other factors, including acidosis, hypoperfusion and hypoxia. The arterial concentration of lactate depends on the rates of its production and use by various organs. Blood lactate concentration is normally maintained < 2 mmol/l, although lactate turnover in healthy resting humans is about 1300 mmol every 24 h. Lactate producers are skeletal muscle, the brain, gut and erythrocytes. Lactate metabolisers are the liver, kidneys and heart. When lactate blood levels exceed 4 mmol/l, the skeletal muscle becomes a net consumer of lactate.

Lactate is a byproduct of glycolysis and is formed in the cytosol catalysed by the enzyme LDH as shown below:

$$Pyruvate + NADH + H^+ = Lactate + NAD^+$$

physiology

This is a reversible reaction that favours lactate synthesis with a lactate:pyruvate ratio that is normally 25:1. Lactate synthesis increases when the rate of pyruvate formation in the cytosol exceeds its rate of use by the mitochondria. This occurs when a rapid increase in metabolic rate occurs or when oxygen delivery to the mitochondria declines, such as in tissue hypoxia. Lactate synthesis may also occur when the rate of glucose metabolism exceeds the oxidative capacity of the mitochondria, as observed with administration of catecholamines or errors of metabolism.

Shock currently is conceptualised as a clinical syndrome resulting from an imbalance between tissue oxygen demands and tissue oxygen supply. Impaired oxygen delivery is the primary problem in hypovolaemic, cardiogenic, distributive (septic) and obstructive (pericardial tamponade, tension pneumothorax) forms of shock. When tissue hypoxia is present, pyruvate oxidation decreases, lactate production increases and ATP formation continues via glycolysis. The amount of lactate produced is believed to correlate with the total oxygen debt, the magnitude of hypoperfusion and the severity of shock. Serial lactate determinations may be helpful in patients resuscitated from shock to assess the adequacy of therapies.

SECTION 3:
PATHOLOGY – ANSWERS

3.1

Answer: B

Metaplasia is a reversible change in which one adult cell type (epithelial or mesenchymal) is replaced by another. It may represent an adaptive substitution of cells that are sensitive to stress by cell types better able to withstand the adverse environment. The most common epithelial metaplasia is columnar to squamous, as occurs in the respiratory tract in response to chronic irritation. In those who are habitual cigarette smokers, the normal ciliated columnar epithelial cells of the trachea and bronchi are often replaced focally or widely by stratified squamous epithelial cells. Stones in the excretory ducts of the salivary glands, pancreas or bile ducts may cause replacement of the normal secretory columnar epithelium by non-functioning stratified squamous epithelium.

However, metaplasia is also seen in connective tissue. Connective tissue metaplasia is the formation of cartilage, bone or adipose tissue (mesenchymal tissues) in tissues that normally do not contain these elements. For example, bone formation in muscle, designated myositis ossificans, occasionally occurs after bone fracture. This type of metaplasia is less clearly seen as an adaptive response. Metaplasia does not result from a change in the phenotype of a differentiated cell type; instead it is the result of a reprogramming of stem cells that are known to exist in normal tissues, or of undifferentiated mesenchymal cells present in connective tissue. In a metaplastic change, these precursor cells differentiate along a new pathway. The differentiation of stem cells to a particular lineage is brought about by signals generated by cytokines, growth factors and extracellular matrix components in the cell's environment. Tissue-specific and differentiation genes are involved in the process, and an increasing number of these are being identified.

3.2

Answer: E

Diabetes exacts a heavy toll on the vascular system. The hallmark of diabetic macrovascular disease is accelerated atherosclerosis involving the aorta and large- and medium-sized arteries. Gangrene is a typical complication of diabetes mellitus with peripheral vascular disease. Gangrene of the lower extremities, as a result of advanced vascular disease, is about 100 times more common in people with diabetes than in the general population. Although gangrenous necrosis is not a distinctive pattern of cell death, the term is still commonly used in surgical clinical practice. It is usually applied to a limb, generally the lower leg, that has lost its blood supply and has undergone coagulation necrosis. When bacterial infection is superimposed, coagulative necrosis is modified by the liquefactive action of the bacteria and the attracted leukocytes (so-called wet gangrene).

A neoplasm is a mass lesion. Coagulopathy, with either thrombosis or haemorrhage, would be more likely to be manifested throughout the body. Coagulopathy is not a feature of diabetes mellitus. Haemosiderin may form locally from remote haemorrhage. With iron overload, it collects in tissues of the mononuclear phagocyte system. Caseation necrosis is a feature of granulomatous inflammation such as tuberculosis (TB). Caseating granulomata are soft, cheesy and white.

3.3

Answer: B

Skeletal muscle is the most likely tissue to resist damage caused by prolonged hypotension because it is the least metabolically active of the ones listed, and also able to function with anaerobic glycolysis. On the other hand, shock can often lead to ischaemic enteritis. The retinal neurons are very sensitive to hypoxia. The myocardium is very active metabolically and is likely to undergo ischaemic damage. Similarly, the neurons of the brain are very sensitive to hypoxia, and the hippocampus in particular.

3.4

Answer: D

Fat necrosis is descriptive of focal areas of fat destruction, typically occurring as a result of release of activated pancreatic lipases into the substance of the pancreas and the peritoneal cavity. This occurs in the calamitous abdominal emergency known as acute pancreatitis. In this disorder, activated pancreatic enzymes escape from acinar cells and ducts, the activated enzymes liquefy fat cell membranes and the activated lipases split the triglyceride esters contained within fat cells. The released fatty acids combine with calcium to produce grossly visible chalky-white areas (fat saponification), which enable the surgeon and the pathologist to identify the lesions. On histological examination, the necrosis takes the form of foci of shadowy outlines of necrotic fat cells, with basophilic calcium deposits, surrounded by an inflammatory reaction.

3.5

Answer: A

Sunburn is a classic example of free radical injury. Free radicals are chemical species that have a single unpaired electron in an outer orbit. Energy created by this unstable configuration is released through reactions with adjacent molecules, such as inorganic or organic chemicals – proteins, lipids, carbohydrates – particularly with key molecules in membranes and nucleic acids. Moreover, free radicals initiate autocatalytic reactions, whereby molecules with which they react are themselves converted into free radicals to propagate the chain of damage. Exposure to ionising radiation or ultraviolet light can hydrolyse water into hydroxyl (OH) and hydrogen (H) free radicals.

3.6

Answer: E

A granuloma is a focus of chronic inflammation consisting of a microscopic aggregation of macrophages that are transformed into epithelium-like cells surrounded by a collar of mononuclear leukocytes, principally lymphocytes and occasionally plasma cells. In the usual haematoxylin and eosin-stained tissue sections, the epithelioid cells have a pale-pink granular cytoplasm with indistinct cell boundaries, often appearing to merge into each other. The nucleus is less dense than that of a lymphocyte, and oval or elongate, and may show folding of the nuclear membrane. Older granulomata develop an enclosing rim of fibroblasts and connective tissue. Frequently, epithelioid cells fuse to form giant cells in the periphery or sometimes in the centre of granulomata. Granulomata are a feature of TB, syphilis, coccidioidomycosis and lepromatous leprosy.

3.7

Answer: D

Type II hypersensitivity is mediated by antibodies directed towards antigens present on cell surfaces or the extracellular matrix. The antigenic determinants may be intrinsic to the cell membrane or matrix, or take the form of an exogenous antigen, such as a drug metabolite, that is adsorbed on a cell surface or matrix. In either case, the hypersensitivity reaction results from the binding of antibodies to normal or altered cell-surface antigens. Examples include autoimmune haemolytic anaemia, autoimmune thrombocytopenic purpura, pemphigus vulgaris, vasculitis caused by ANCA (antibody to neutrophil cytoplasmic antigens), acute rheumatic fever, myasthenia gravis, insulin-resistant diabetes, pernicious anaemia and Graves' disease (hyperthyroidism).

3.8

Answer: A

Hypersensitivity reaction to penicillin is a classic example of a type I hypersensitivity reaction. Immediate, or type I, hypersensitivity is a rapidly developing immunological reaction occurring within minutes after the combination of an antigen to an antibody bound to mast cells in individuals previously sensitised to the antigen. These reactions are often called an allergy, and the antigens that elicit them are allergens. Immediate hypersensitivity may occur as a systemic disorder or a local reaction. The systemic reaction usually follows

pathology

injection of an antigen to which the host has become sensitised. Often within minutes a state of shock is produced, which is sometimes fatal. The nature of local reactions varies depending on the portal of entry of the allergen and may take the form of localised cutaneous swellings (skin allergy, hives), nasal and conjunctival discharge (allergic rhinitis and conjunctivitis), hay fever, bronchial asthma or allergic gastroenteritis (food allergy).

3.9

Answer: A

Metaplasia is the substitution of one tissue normally found at a site for another. It is a reversible change. Epithelial metaplasia is a two-edged sword and, in most circumstances, represents an undesirable change. Moreover, the influences that predispose to metaplasia, if persistent, may induce malignant transformation in metaplastic epithelium. Metaplasia from squamous to columnar type is seen in Barrett's oesophagus, in which the oesophageal squamous epithelium is replaced by intestinal-like columnar cells under the influence of refluxed gastric acid. The epithelium undergoes metaplasia in response to the ongoing inflammation from reflux of gastric contents. It is common in the lower oesophagus with gastro-oesophageal reflux disease (GORD). Cancers may arise in these areas, and these are typically glandular (adeno)carcinomas.

The growth of the epithelial cells must become disordered in order to be dysplastic. Hyperplasia may occur with inflammation, as the number of cells increases, but hyperplasia does not explain the presence of the columnar cells. A carcinoma has the cellular atypia with hyperchromatism and pleomorphism. Goblet cells would not be seen. Ischaemia would be unusual at this site and would be marked by coagulative necrosis.

3.10

Answer: D

Hypernatraemia results from one of two basic mechanisms: water is lost and not adequately replaced or, less commonly, too much salt is

pathology

taken in with insufficient water. Electrolyte-free water can be lost as pure water, with no accompanying electrolyte, or it can be lost in hypotonic fluids, which have lower electrolyte concentrations than plasma. Hypotonic losses can be thought of as mixtures of isotonic fluid and free water. Pure water and hypotonic fluid losses, the most common causes of hypernatraemia, are typically associated with a contracted extracellular fluid (ECF) volume. However, this is not always the case. When hypernatraemia is caused by a rapid intake of salt (acute salt poisoning), the extracellular volume expands because of water drawn from the intracellular space. In critically ill patients, extracellular volume expansion with oedema often coexists with hypernatraemia; the finding reflects free water losses in patients who become oedematous after fluid resuscitation for shock or underlying conditions such as congestive heart failure, renal disease and hepatic cirrhosis.

Faecal losses of water contain electrolytes at a concentration comparable to that of plasma, except when osmotic cathartics such as sorbitol or lactulose are given. These cathartic agents osmotically attract electrolyte-free water to the intestinal lumen, leading to hypotonic fluid losses. Oral sorbitol is a non-absorbable solute, given with sodium polystyrene sulphonate to treat hyperkalaemia or with charcoal to treat poisoning; the sorbitol osmotically attracts electrolyte-free water into the intestinal lumen, where it is eliminated in the stool. Similarly, lactulose, which is used to treat hepatic encephalopathy, can promote large electrolyte-free water losses, causing a high incidence of hypernatraemia unless the lost water is replaced.

3.11

Answer: C

Haemosiderin is a haemoglobin-derived, golden-yellow–brown, granular or crystalline pigment, in which form iron is stored in cells. Iron is normally carried by specific transport proteins – the transferrins. In cells, it is stored in association with a protein, apoferritin, to form ferritin micelles. Ferritin is a constituent of most cell types. When there is a local or systemic excess of iron, ferritin forms haemosiderin granules, which are easily seen with the light microscope. Thus, haemosiderin pigment represents aggregates of ferritin micelles. Under normal conditions, small amounts of haemosiderin can be seen in the mononuclear phagocytes of the bone marrow, spleen and liver, all actively engaged in red cell breakdown.

Excesses of iron cause haemosiderin to accumulate within cells, as either a localised process or a systemic derangement. Local excesses of iron and haemosiderin result from gross haemorrhages or the myriad minute haemorrhages that accompany severe vascular congestion. The best example of localised haemosiderosis is the common bruise. After local haemorrhage, the area is at first red–blue. With lysis of the erythrocytes, the haemoglobin eventually undergoes transformation to haemosiderin. Macrophages take part in this process by phagocytosing the red cell debris, and then lysosomal enzymes eventually convert the haemoglobin, through a sequence of pigments, into haemosiderin. The play of colours through which the bruise passes reflects these transformations. The original red–blue colour of haemoglobin is transformed to varying shades of green blue, comprising the local formation of biliverdin (green bile), then bilirubin (red bile) and, thereafter, the iron moiety of haemoglobin is deposited as golden-yellow haemosiderin.

Lipofuchsin is a 'wear-and-tear' pigment that builds up in cells of tissues (such as the myocardium and liver) over many years. Melanin pigment darkens the skin as its concentrations increase from sunlight exposure (tanning). A generalised yellow colour, jaundice, can be the result of hyperbilirubinaemia. Glycogen is stored in striated muscle and liver and imparts no grossly visible colour change.

3.12

Answer: B

The total parenteral nutrition (TPN) solution must be more concentrated for patients who require fluid restriction (eg those with pulmonary and cardiac failure). A litre of concentrated TPN solution usually contains a combination of 500 ml $D_{60}W$ or $D_{70}W$ and 500 ml of 10% or 15% amino acids plus additives. Patients in renal failure (serum creatinine > 2 mg/dl) who cannot be dialysed and require fluid restriction should receive a special renal failure TPN solution. Each litre

pathology

of solution contains a combination of 500 ml $D_{60}W$ or $D_{70}W$ and just 500 ml essential amino acids plus limited amounts of sodium, potassium, magnesium and phosphate. Patients in renal failure who can undergo dialysis should receive a TPN solution that contains 500 ml $D_{60}W$ or $D_{70}W$ and 500 ml of 8.5% standard amino acids (a combination of essential and non-essential) plus additives, with limited amounts of sodium, potassium, magnesium and phosphate.

Hepatic encephalopathy has been related to the high levels of aromatic amino acids (phenylalanine, tyrosine and tryptophan) in the plasma, acting as precursors of false neurotransmitters (amines) in the central and peripheral nervous systems. Administration of branched-chain amino acid solution (enriched with leucine, isoleucine and valine) will normalise the plasma aminogram and possibly reverse the coma in patients with chronic encephalopathy. Glucose should be used as a source of energy in hepatic failure but it needs careful monitoring. Blood levels may fluctuate widely because carbohydrate tolerance is impaired as a result of peripheral insulin resistance. Intravenous lipid infusions are contraindicated because they have a synergistic effect in producing coma, particularly with ammonia, and they may exacerbate coma by displacing tryptophan from plasma protein-binding sites. Administration of high doses of glucose to patients with borderline respiratory function may increase their carbon dioxide production to the point of compromising respiratory function. Such patients may benefit from the replacement of some glucose energy intake with fat. High rates of infusion of amino acids may increase respiratory drive in some patients; this may be important therapeutically.

3.13

Answer: B

Morphine is contraindicated in patients with head injury as a result of its property of raising the intracranial pressure. A serious action is stoppage of respiratory exchange in emphysema or cor pulmonale. Hence, it is contraindicated in patients with chronic obstructive pulmonary disease (COPD). Patients with adrenal insufficiency or myxoedema may experience extended and increased effects from opioids. Morphine is mainly metabolised by the liver, hence it should be avoided in patients with liver disease. Morphine is the analgesic of choice for relieving pain associated with acute myocardial infarction.

3.14

Answer: D

The principal difference between thermal burns and chemical burns is that in chemical burns tissue destruction continues as long as contact is maintained, unless the agent is inactivated by its reaction with the tissues. This means that chemical burns are usually deeper than they initially appear and progress with time. The initial treatment of a chemical burn is dilution of the chemical with water. This is best delivered by continuous running water or by prolonged hydrotherapy in large volume tanks for 12 h. Neutralising agents should not be used because they cause exothermic reactions and increased tissue damage.

3.15

Answer: C

The bladder ruptures extraperitoneally as a result of perforations by adjacent bony fragments from the site of pelvic fracture. Disruption of the urethra is often a result of straddle injury. A delayed repair of the extraperitoneal rupture may be required once the retroperitoneal bleeding has been controlled and the condition of the patient stabilised. These patients are at very high risk of haemorrhagic complications associated with dissection into the retroperitoneal pelvic haematoma.

3.16

Answer: C

The retroperitoneal location of the pancreas precludes the early development of peritonitis. Diagnostic peritoneal lavage will not be helpful except in the most extensive injury where there is transudation of retroperitoneal blood in the peritoneal cavity. Computed tomography (CT) is an excellent technique for evaluation

pathology

of patients with suspected injuries to the pancreas. A progressive rise in the amylase over the first 24–48 h of hospitalisation is strongly suggestive of injury to either the pancreas or the duodenum. Ductal transection in the neck, body or tail is an indication of distal pancreatectomy or roux-en-Y distal pancreatojejunostomy. Pancreatic fistulae originating exclusively from the parenchyma exclusively of the main duct in the body or head will usually close spontaneously.

3.17

Answer: C

Non-surgical management of stable patients with hepatic injuries diagnosed on CT is now practised in many centres. CT criteria for non-operative management include the following:

1. Simple hepatic parenchymal laceration or intrahepatic haematomas
2. No evidence of active bleeding
3. Intraperitoneal blood loss < 250 ml
4. An absence of other intraperitoneal injuries requiring operation.

Associated splenic trauma is an indication for surgical intervention.

3.18

Answer: A

Since the first descriptions of diagnostic peritoneal lavage/tap (DPL) by Root and colleagues in the mid-1960s, this technique has remained a mainstay of the evaluation of the patient with possible intra-abdominal injuries after blunt trauma. Patients in whom this technique should be considered are listed as follows:

1. A patient with an altered sensorium from a head injury, drug ingestion or alcohol intoxication.
2. A patient with altered sensation such as from a spinal

cord injury.

3.   A patient with injury to adjacent structures such as the ribs or transverse processes of the vertebrae.
4.   The patient with equivocal findings on physical examination of the abdomen.

The absolute contraindication to the technique is an obvious indication for laparotomy. Relative contraindications include scars on the abdominal wall reflecting previous intra-abdominal operations, the latter stages of pregnancy, morbid obesity, a coagulopathy and significant haematomas of the abdominal wall related to pelvic fractures.

3.19

Answer: C

In addition to the profound glucose flow, there is profound insulin insensitivity. These effects do not occur because of inadequate quantities of insulin released from the endocrine pancreas, because in most cases there is hyperinsulinaemia. However, the cause for the marked insulin resistance is related to diminished food intake and an altered hormonal environment – the counterregulatory hormones glucagon, cortisol and catecholamines – that exert anti-insulin activity. In the initial phase of injury, blood volume is reduced, peripheral resistance increases and cardiac output falls. Marked vasodilatation occurs in vessels that perfuse injured areas and this is accompanied by the ingrowth of new capillaries. Control of wound circulation is similar to other critical tissues (heart, brain, working skeletal muscle), in which blood flow varies as a function of local metabolic conditions rather than being part of integrated central vasoregulatory reflexes. This means that, as long as blood pressure is maintained, wound perfusion is ensured. Muscle is the origin of the nitrogen loss in the urine after extensive injury. However, it has been recognised that the composition of amino acid efflux from skeletal muscle does not reflect the composition of muscle protein. Alanine and glutamine constitute the majority of amino acids released, whereas each makes up only about 6% of muscle protein.

pathology

3.20

Answer: B

Zone I injuries occur at the base of the neck and do not allow easy accessibility from an operative standpoint. Injuries in zone I may involve proximal carotid, subclavian or innominate vessels, and patients are at risk of exsanguinating haemorrhage, which may be occult if the blood tracks into the chest or mediastinum. Thoracic inlet injuries must therefore be investigated with panendoscopy and arteriography. Zone II injuries are midneck injuries (from the clavicular heads to angles of the jaw). Injuries that occur above the angle of the mandible (zone III) may involve the petrous or cavernous portions of the internal carotid artery, the vertebral artery or deep branches of the external carotid artery. Wide exposure of this area and distal vascular control may be difficult to obtain.

Routine exploration as a diagnostic manoeuvre may be both hazardous and inaccurate. Gunshot wounds account for most of these injuries, and patients may present with haematoma or haemorrhage from the mouth, nose, throat or wound. There are often associated neurological injuries. Arteriography is the diagnostic method of choice for zone III injuries. It has proved highly sensitive and specific, and a negative study obviates the need for vascular exploration. Moreover, therapeutic embolisation may be indicated for inaccessible branches of the external carotid artery, the vertebral artery or a thrombosed internal carotid in a comatose patient. Zone III or upper neck injuries (above the angle of the jaw) prompt arteriography before any needed exploration. CT is a particularly useful diagnostic tool for suspected laryngeal fracture or penetrating laryngeal injury.

3.21

Answer: C

The features are suggestive of thrombophlebitis. The deep leg veins account for more than 90% of cases of thrombophlebitis and phlebothrombosis, two designations for inflammation and venous thrombosis. Cardiac failure, neoplasia, pregnancy, obesity, the postoperative state and prolonged bedrest or immobilisation are the most important clinical predispositions. Genetic hypercoagulability syndromes can also be associated with venous thrombosis.

Septic emboli produce focal haemorrhage or infarction and are usually arterial. The peripheral oedema that accompanies congestive heart failure would be symmetrical. Cellulitis would produce a warm, swollen, tender appearance from the subcutaneous inflammation. Infarction is a focal process from arterial occlusion.

3.22

Answer: D

Immobilisation after fracture, particularly in elderly people, is a significant risk for development of deep venous thrombosis, followed by pulmonary embolism. Pulmonary embolism is a common and serious clinical sequel to deep leg vein thrombosis. The contraction of surrounding muscles tends to 'milk' the contents loose from their attachments to the vein walls. Not infrequently, the first manifestation of thrombophlebitis is the development of an embolic episode; in a very ill patient pulmonary embolisation often constitutes the final blow.

Older people are at risk of cancer, but the course of events in this clinical vignette suggests immobilisation leading to pulmonary thromboembolism. Similarly signs and symptoms of an infectious disease such as TB were not present. Elderly people are at risk of pneumonia when in hospital; however, signs and symptoms of an infection mark the course, which is not the case in this scenario. Congestive heart failure is a possibility in elderly people, but in the setting given is unlikely to be the cause of the sudden death.

3.23

Answer: E

The clinical picture suggests marked blood loss with shock. There will be vasoconstriction in the skin in response to the hypovolaemia. Decreased renal blood flow from shock can lead to acute tubular necrosis. The lack of tissue perfusion with shock leads to increased anaerobic glycolysis and lactic acidosis. The clinical significance of haemorrhage depends on the volume and rate of bleeding. Rapid loss of up to 20% of the blood volume or slow losses of even larger amounts may have little impact in healthy adults; greater losses may, however, result in haemorrhagic (hypovolaemic) shock. The site of haemorrhage is also important; bleeding that would be trivial in the subcutaneous tissues may cause death if located in the brain because the skull is unyielding and bleeding there can result in increased intracranial pressure and herniation.

Finally, loss of iron and subsequent iron-deficiency anaemia become a consideration in chronic or recurrent external blood loss (eg peptic ulcer or menstrual bleeding). In contrast, when red cells are retained, as in haemorrhage into body cavities or tissues, the iron can be reused for haemoglobin synthesis.

This patient has signs of marked blood loss, so his haematocrit should be low – probably in the 20s or lower. Hypoglycaemia is not a feature of blood loss with shock. The patient has had blood loss, but the oxygen-carrying capacity of the remaining red blood cells (RBCs) is not affected, and his ability to oxygenate is not completely lost. An elevated troponin I suggests myocardial ischaemia. With good coronary blood flow in a young person, the myocardium is not seriously affected until the patient is near death.

3.24

Answer: B

The brightness on the radiograph suggests calcification from the osseous metaplasia that developed in the healing process. This condition is known as myositis ossificans, because there is bone formation in the injured muscle. Connective tissue metaplasia is the formation of cartilage, bone or adipose tissue (mesenchymal tissues) in tissues that normally do not contain these elements. This type of metaplasia is less clearly seen as an adaptive response.

Dysplasia refers to disordered epithelial cell growth. There are increased numbers of cells in this exaggerated healing process, but this does not account for the bright calcification. Although some cells may increase in size, the process is one of bone formation – metaplastic bone formation as part of an exaggerated healing process, not the uncontrolled growth of a neoplasm.

3.25

Answer: A

Neurofibroma arises from the connective tissue of the nerve sheath. The 'painful' subcutaneous nodule forms a smooth firm swelling that may be moved in a lateral direction, but is otherwise fixed by the nerve from which it arises. As the nerve fibres are 'part and parcel' of the tumour, they are difficult to remove without the removal of the nerve itself. In major nerves recurrence is a problem, as is malignant (sarcomatous) change. Plexiform neurofibromatosis is a rare condition characterised by enormous thickening of the affected nerve as a result of myxofibromatous degeneration of the endoneurium. This rare condition usually occurs in connection with branches of the fifth cranial nerve, although it may occur in the extremities. Von Recklinghausen's disease of the nerves is an autosomal dominant disease in which any cranial, spinal or peripheral nerve may be diffusely or nodularly thickened. Associated pigmentation is common.

3.26

Answer: C

In permeation the malignant cells grow along the lymphatic vessels from the primary growth. This may occur even in a retrograde direction. The cancer cells stimulate perilymphatic fibrosis, but this does not stop the advance of the disease. In some instances, notably malignant melanoma, groups of cells may so overcome the surrounding fibrosis that they give rise to intermediate deposits between the primary growth and the lymph nodes. Malignant melanoma spreads by permeation as well as embolism. In embolism cancer cells that invade a lymphatic vessel can break away and are carried by the lymph circulation to a regional node, so that nodes comparatively distant from the tumour may be involved in the early stages. Another example, of 'kiss cancer', is carcinoma of the lower lip affecting the upper. For the abdomen, transcoelomic spread is especially notable when cells from a colloid carcinoma of the stomach gravitate on to an active ovary and give rise to malignant ovarian tumours (Krukenberg's tumour). A rodent ulcer (synonymous with basal cell carcinoma) is a locally malignant tumour; distant metastasis via the lymphatics or haematogenous spread is virtually non-existent.

pathology

3.27

Answer: E

Trophic ulcers (*trophe*, Greek for nutrition) are caused by an impairment of the nutrition of the tissues, which depends on an adequate blood supply and also a properly functioning nerve supply. Ischaemia and anaesthesia will therefore cause these ulcers. Thus, in the arm, chronic vasospasm and syringomyelia will cause ulceration of the tips of the fingers (respectively painful and painless). In the leg, painful ischaemic ulcers occur around the ankle or on the dorsum of the foot. Neuropathic ulcers caused by anaesthesia (diabetic neuritis, spina bifida, tabes dorsalis, leprosy or a peripheral nerve injury) are often called perforating ulcers. Starting in a corn or bunion, they penetrate the foot, and suppuration may involve the bones and joints and spread along fascial planes upwards, even involving the calf.

3.28

Answer: C

Marjolin's ulcer is a carcinoma that develops in a scar. Chronic wounds and scar tissues are prone to an increased risk of skin cancer. In 1828, Jean-Nicholas Marjolin described the occurrence of tumours in post-traumatic scar tissue. Marjolin's ulcer most frequently occurs in old burn scars, but it has also been reported in relation to osteomyelitis, frostbite, venous stasis ulcers, skin graft donor sites, chronic decubitus ulcers, gunshot wounds, puncture wounds, dog bites, occult trauma, injection sites and scar tissue around colostomies. In adults the usual time for the appearance of carcinoma in scar tissue is around the age of 53–59 years. As a general rule, the latency period between the burn injury and the appearance of cancer is 25–40 years. It grows slowly, because the scar is relatively avascular. It is painless because the tissue contains no nerves. Secondary deposits do not occur in the regional lymph nodes because lymphatic vessels have been destroyed. If the ulcer invades normal tissue surrounding the scar, it extends at a normal rate, and lymph nodes are then liable to be involved.

3.29

Answer: D

Persistence of a sinus or fistula is the result of one of the following:

- A foreign body or necrotic tissue is present, eg a suture, hairs, a sequestrum, a faecolith or even a worm (as in guinea-worm infestation).
- Inefficient or non-dependent drainage: a long, narrow, tortuous track predisposes to inefficient drainage.
- Unrelieved obstruction of the lumen of a viscus or tube distal to the fistula.
- Absence of rest, such as occurs in fistula *in ano*, caused by the normal contractions of the sphincter that also force faecal matter into the internal opening.
- The walls have become lined with epithelium or endothelium (arteriovenous fistula).
- Dense fibrosis prevents contraction and healing.
- Type of infection, eg TB or actinomycosis.
- The presence of malignant disease.
- Persistent discharge, such as urine, faeces or cerebrospinal fluid (CSF).
- Ischaemia.
- Drugs, eg steroids.
- Malnutrition.
- Interference, eg artefacts.
- Irradiation, eg rectovaginal fistula after treatment for carcinoma of the cervix.

3.30

Answer: B

Xeroderma pigmentosum is an autosomal recessive disorder characterised by failure of DNA-repair mechanisms. There is a markedly increased incidence of skin cancers in xeroderma pigmentosum. Ultraviolet light is thought to enhance neoplastic change in the skin by dimer formation between neighbouring thymine pairs in DNA. These deleterious changes in DNA are repaired by enzymatically mediated mechanisms. In xeroderma pigmentosum, specific enzyme deficiencies result in failure of such repair and a consequent increase in the tumorigenic effect of sunlight.

pathology

3.31

Answer: A

Granuloma formation with TB is a classic type IV hypersensitivity reaction. The cell-mediated type of hypersensitivity is initiated by antigen-activated (sensitised) T lymphocytes. It includes the delayed-type hypersensitivity reactions mediated by CD4+ T cells, and direct cell cytotoxicity mediated by CD8+ T cells. It is the principal pattern of immunological response not only to a variety of intracellular microbiological agents, such as *Mycobacterium tuberculosis*, but also to many viruses, fungi, protozoa and parasites. So-called contact skin sensitivity to chemical agents and graft rejection are other instances of cell-mediated reactions. In addition, many autoimmune diseases are now known to be caused by T-cell-mediated reactions.

Type I reactions are associated with allergy and anaphylaxis. Type II reactions are associated with complement-mediated immune reactions. Graft-versus-host disease (GVHD) does not produce a granulomatous reaction. Granulomatous reactions are based mainly on cell-mediated immunity.

3.32

Answer: B

This is a type I hypersensitivity reaction with systemic anaphylaxis, in part mediated by the most important vasoactive amine – histamine. About 20% of people will have some reaction to penicillin or similar drugs, and a few of these will be severe. Histamine causes intense smooth muscle contraction, increased vascular permeability, and increased secretion by nasal, bronchial and gastric glands.

Interleukin-1 (IL-1) is more involved with the appearance of fever with inflammation. Bradykinin mediates the appearance of pain and vascular permeability. Complement C5a is a chemotactic factor. Thromboxane, generated by the cyclo-oxygenase pathway of arachidonic acid metabolism, mediates platelet aggregation and vasoconstriction to promote haemostasis.

3.33

Answer: C

Fibroblast growth factor (FGF) can stimulate all aspects of angiogenesis. This is a family of growth factors containing more than ten members, of which acidic FGF (aFGF, or FGF-1) and basic FGF (bFGF, or FGF-2) are the best characterised. FGF-1 and FGF-2 are made by a variety of cells. Released FGFs associate with heparan sulphate in the extracellular matrix, which can serve as a reservoir for storing inactive factors. FGFs are recognised by a family of cell-surface receptors that have intrinsic tyrosine kinase activity. A large number of functions are attributed to FGFs, including the following:

- New blood vessel formation (angiogenesis): FGF-2, in particular, has the ability to induce the steps necessary for new blood vessel formation both in vivo and in vitro (see below).
- Wound repair: FGFs participate in macrophage, fibroblast and endothelial cell migration in damaged tissues and migration of epithelium to form new epidermis.
- Development: FGFs play a role in skeletal muscle development and lung maturation, eg FGF-6 and its receptor induce myoblast proliferation and suppress myocyte differentiation, providing a supply of proliferating myocytes. FGF-2 is also thought to be involved in the generation of angioblasts during embryogenesis. FGF-1 and FGF-2 are involved in the specification of the liver from endodermal cells.
- Haematopoiesis: FGFs have been implicated in the differentiation of specific lineages of blood cells and development of bone marrow stroma.

Platelet-derived growth factor (PDGF) released from macrophages as well as activated platelets can stimulate fibroblast growth for collagen synthesis. Phospholipases aid in stimulation of intracellular protein kinases, which promote protein phosphorylation. Fibronectin is a component of the extracellular matrix that helps to link cells together. Epidermal growth factor (EGF) is a stimulator of cell growth through activation of tyrosine kinases in the cells; it can also stimulate angiogenesis to a degree.

pathology

3.34

Answer: C

At 3 months about 70–80% of the tensile strength of non-wounded skin is reached, which is about as much as will be obtained. After 3 months, there will be little gain in tensile strength. When the sutures are removed, usually at the end of the first week, wound strength is about 10% that of unwounded skin, but strength increases rapidly over the next 4 weeks. This rate of increase then slows at approximately the third month after the original incision, and reaches a plateau at about 70–80% of the tensile strength of unwounded skin, a condition that may persist for life. The recovery of tensile strength results from the excess of collagen synthesis over collagen degradation during the first 2 months of healing, and, at later times, from structural modifications of collagen fibres (cross-linking, increased fibre size) after collagen synthesis ceases. At 1 week the wound site has granulation tissue, but little collagen at this point. At 1 month collagen is being laid down, but a plateau phase has not been reached.

3.35

Answer: C

Some people have an inappropriate wound healing response with excessive collagenisation. Excessive formation of the components of the repair process can also complicate wound healing. Aberrations of growth may occur even in what may begin initially as normal wound healing. The accumulation of excessive amounts of collagen may give rise to a raised scar known as a hypertrophic scar; if the scar tissue grows beyond the boundaries of the original wound and does not regress, it is called a keloid. Keloid formation appears to be an individual predisposition, and for unknown reasons this aberration is somewhat more common in African–American individuals. The mechanisms of keloid formation are still unknown. Another deviation in wound healing is the formation of excessive amounts of granulation tissue, which protrudes above the level of the surrounding skin and blocks re-epithelialisation. This has been called exuberant granulation (or, with more literary fervour, proud flesh). Excessive granulation must be removed by cautery or surgical excision to permit restoration of the continuity of the epithelium. Finally (fortunately rarely), incisional scars or traumatic injuries may be followed by exuberant proliferation of fibroblasts and other connective tissue elements that may, in fact, recur after excision. Called desmoids, or aggressive fibromatoses, these lie in the interface between benign proliferations and malignant (although low-grade) tumours.

The wound will not have excessive collagen with poor wound healing. Sutures can produce small foreign body granulomata that typically are not visible. Trauma does not lead to neoplasia, so fibrosarcoma is the least likely to be seen in this case. A wound infection will produce dehiscence and abscess formation that delays or disrupts collagenisation.

3.36

Answer: B

Liposarcomas are one of the most common sarcomas of adulthood and appear in those in their 40s to 60s; they are uncommon in children. They usually arise in the deep soft tissues of the proximal extremities and retroperitoneum and are notorious for developing into large tumours. Histologically, liposarcomas can be divided into well-differentiated, myxoid, round cell and pleomorphic variants. The well-differentiated variant is relatively indolent, the myxoid type is intermediate in its malignant behaviour, and the round cell and pleomorphic variants are usually aggressive and frequently metastasise. All types of liposarcoma recur locally and often repeatedly unless adequately excised.

Melanomas arise on the skin in most cases and are rarely visceral or in soft tissue. A hamartoma is a peculiar small benign neoplasm composed of tissues normal to a site, but just in a jumbled mass. A pulmonary hamartoma is the most common of these. Adenocarcinomas do not arise in soft tissues. Sarcomas arise in soft tissues. Finally, it is unlikely that matted nodes with lymphoma would reach this size.

pathology

3.37

Answer: E

The outcome for women with breast cancer varies widely. Some women have the same life expectancy as women without breast cancer. Other women have only a 13% chance of being alive in 5 years. Except for the few women (< 10%) with distant metastases at presentation or with inflammatory carcinoma, prognosis is determined by the pathological examination of the primary carcinoma and the axillary lymph nodes. This information is important for counselling patients about the likely outcome of their disease, choosing appropriate treatment and accurately classifying groups of similar patients for clinical trials. Aneuploidy is a bad prognostic sign because such neoplastic cells tend to be much less differentiated and much more aggressive.

The presence of oestrogen receptors suggests better differentiation and the possibility of treatment with hormonal agents. Well-differentiated tumours usually have a better prognosis. Intraductal growth suggests that this carcinoma remains *in situ*; infiltration indicates a more aggressive behaviour. The stage $T_1 N_0 M_0$ is the lowest possible stage for any tumour. Neoplasms with a low stage tend to be less aggressive and have a better prognosis.

3.38

Answer: A

Hashimoto's thyroiditis (or chronic lymphocytic thyroiditis) is the most common cause of hypothyroidism in areas of the world where iodine levels are sufficient. It is characterised by gradual thyroid failure because of autoimmune destruction of the thyroid gland. The name Hashimoto's thyroiditis is derived from the 1912 report by Hashimoto describing patients with goitre and intense lymphocytic infiltration of the thyroid (struma lymphomatosa). This disorder is most prevalent at the ages between 45 and 65 years and is more common in women than in men, with a female predominance of 10–20:1. Although it is primarily a disease of older women, it can occur in children and is a major cause of non-endemic goitre in children.

pathology

Hashimoto's thyroiditis is an autoimmune disease in which the immune system reacts against a variety of thyroid antigens. The overriding feature of Hashimoto's thyroiditis is progressive depletion of thyroid epithelial cells (thyrocytes), which are gradually replaced by mononuclear cell infiltration and fibrosis. Multiple immunological mechanisms may contribute to the death of thyrocytes. Sensitisation of autoreactive CD4+ T-helper cells to thyroid antigens appears to be the initiating event. Anti-thyroid autoantibodies are helpful in establishing the diagnosis.

Subacute granulomatous thyroiditis (DeQuervain's disease) leads to transient thyroid enlargement with pain, but the course runs for a month or two and patients typically do not become hypothyroid. Carcinomas of the thyroid are not typically associated with autoantibodies. Medullary carcinomas are characterised by secretion of calcitonin and usually seen as a component of multiple endocrine neoplasia (MEN). Graves' disease produces hyperthyroidism and thyroid enlargement. Removal of the thyroid as a treatment can lead to hypothyroidism.

3.39

Answer: C

She most probably has osteoporosis with accelerated bone loss, leading to the propensity for fractures. Physical inactivity further accelerates bone loss and decreases muscle mass and agility, which contributes to falls. Osteoporosis is a disease characterised by increased porosity of the skeleton as a result of reduced bone mass. The associated structural changes predispose the bone to fracture. The disorder may be localised to a certain bone or region, as in disuse osteoporosis of a limb, or involve the entire skeleton, as a manifestation of a metabolic bone disease. Generalised osteoporosis may be primary or secondary to a large variety of conditions. The most common forms of osteoporosis are senile and postmenopausal osteoporosis. In these disorders, the critical loss of bone mass makes the skeleton vulnerable to fractures.

An osteomyelitis is not typical at this age and does not usually present as fractures in multiple locations. Osteogenesis imperfecta, an inherited disorder of collagen synthesis, is initially diagnosed in

pathology

fetuses and young children. Polyostotic fibrous dysplasia is a rare disorder that can be seen with McCune–Albright syndrome. A so-called 'pathological fracture' can occur from weakening of the bone by metastases, but such patients are often very ill, with a history of weight loss and prior bone pain.

3.40

Answer: E

A 'small round blue cell' tumour of bone is Ewing's sarcoma, commonly seen at this age. Ewing's sarcoma accounts for approximately 6–10% of primary malignant bone tumours and follows osteosarcoma as the second most common group of bone sarcomas in children. Of all bone sarcomas, Ewing's sarcoma has the youngest average age at presentation, because most patients are 10–15 years old, and about 80% are younger than 20 years. Boys are affected slightly more frequently than girls, and there is a striking predilection for white individuals; black individuals are rarely afflicted. In about 85% of Ewing's sarcomas, there is a t(11;22)(q24;q12) translocation; in 5–10% of cases, the translocation is t(21;21)(q21;q12), and in less than 1% of tumours a t(7;22)(q22;12) translocation is present.

Arising in the medullary cavity, Ewing's sarcoma usually invades the cortex and periosteum, producing a soft-tissue mass. The tumour is tan-white and frequently contains areas of haemorrhage and necrosis. It is composed of sheets of uniform, small, round cells that are slightly larger than lymphocytes. Ewing's sarcoma usually arises in the diaphyses of long tubular bones, especially the femur and the flat bones of the pelvis. They present as painful enlarging masses, and the affected site is frequently tender, warm and swollen. Some patients have systemic findings, including fever, elevated sedimentation rate, anaemia and leukocytosis, which mimic infection. Plain radiographs show a destructive lytic tumour that has permeative margins and extension into the surrounding soft tissues. The characteristic periosteal reaction produces layers of reactive bone deposited in an onion-skin fashion.

Medulloblastoma, although composed of small blue cells, arises in the CNS (posterior fossa) in children. Although a neuroblastoma is composed of small blue cells, it typically arises in the adrenals in children.

A chondroblastoma arises in the epiphysis of bone. An osteoblastoma is essentially just a large osteoid osteoma, often in vertebrae.

3.41

Answer: D

Osteoid production is characteristic for osteosarcoma, which is defined as a malignant mesenchymal tumour in which the cancerous cells produce bone matrix. It is the most common primary malignant tumour of bone, exclusive of myeloma and lymphoma, and accounts for about 20% of primary bone cancers. Osteosarcoma occurs in all age groups but has a bimodal age distribution; 75% occur in patients younger than 20. The smaller second peak occurs in elderly people, who frequently suffer from conditions known to be associated with the development of osteosarcoma – Paget's disease, bone infarcts and prior irradiation. Overall, men are more commonly affected than women (1.6:1). The tumours usually arise in the metaphyseal region of the long bones of the extremities, and almost 60% occur around the knee. Any bone may be involved, however, and in those aged over 25 the incidence in flat bones and long bones is almost equal.

Metastases are unlikely to occur at this age. Overall, metastases are the most common malignancy involving bone. Primary bone tumours are not common. Ewing's sarcoma has a peak incidence at a younger age, and most often involves the diaphyseal region. It does not produce osteoid. Chondrosarcomas do not make osteoid. They can occur over a wide age range. Myelomas are seen in older adults and produce lytic bone lesions filled with plasma cells.

3.42

Answer: C

Longitudinal tears in the oesophagus at the oesophagogastric junction or gastric cardia are termed 'Mallory–Weiss tears' and are believed to be the consequence of severe retching or vomiting. They are encountered most commonly in people with alcohol problems, in whom they are attributed to episodes of excessive vomiting in the setting of an alcoholic stupor. Normally, a reflex relaxation of the musculature of the gastrointestinal (GI) tract precedes the anti-peristaltic wave of contraction. During episodes of prolonged vomiting, it is speculated that this reflex relaxation fails to occur. The refluxing gastric contents suddenly overwhelm the contraction of the musculature at the gastric inlet, and massive dilatation with tearing of the stretched wall ensues. As these tears may occur in people who have no history of vomiting or alcoholism, there must be other mechanisms; underlying hiatal hernia is a known predisposing factor. Oesophageal lacerations account for 5–10% of bleeding episodes in the upper GI tract.

Most often, bleeding is not profuse and ceases without surgical intervention, although massive haematemesis may occur. Supportive therapy, such as vasoconstrictive medications and transfusions, and sometimes balloon tamponade, is usually all that is required. Healing tends to be prompt, with minimal to no residua. The rare instance of oesophageal rupture is known as Boerhaave's syndrome and may be a catastrophic event. Oesophageal variceal bleeding should also be suspected with such a history.

Diverticula of the oesophagus do not often bleed. Typical symptoms include dysphagia, food regurgitation and a mass in the neck; aspiration with resultant pneumonia is a significant risk. Barrett's mucosa is associated with reflux with inflammation and possible ulceration, but bleeding is not usually massive. There may be reflux along with inflammation and possible ulceration, but bleeding is not typically massive.

3.43

Answer: B

Chronic gastritis is defined as the presence of chronic mucosal inflammatory changes leading eventually to mucosal atrophy and intestinal metaplasia, usually in the absence of erosions. The epithelial changes may become dysplastic and constitute a background for the development of carcinoma. Chronic gastritis is notable for distinct causal subgroups and patterns of histological alterations that vary in different parts of the world. In the western world, the prevalence of histological changes indicative of chronic gastritis in the later decades of life is higher than 50%. By far the most important aetiological association with chronic gastritis is chronic infection by the bacillus *Helicobacter pylori*.

Zollinger and Ellison first called attention to the association of pancreatic islet cell lesions with hypersecretion of gastric acid and severe peptic ulceration, which are present in 90–95% of patients. In the Zollinger–Ellison syndrome, hypergastrinaemia from a pancreatic or duodenal tumour stimulates extreme gastric acid secretion, which in turn causes peptic ulceration. The duodenal and gastric ulcers are often multiple; although they are identical to those found in the general population, they are often unresponsive to the usual modalities of therapy. In addition, ulcers may also occur in unusual locations such as the jejunum; when intractable jejunal ulcers are found, the Zollinger–Ellison syndrome should be considered. More than 50% of the patients have diarrhoea; in 30%, it is the presenting symptom. This syndrome is rare.

In pernicious anaemia the changes in the stomach are those of diffuse chronic gastritis. The most characteristic histological alteration is the atrophy of the fundic glands, affecting both chief cells and parietal cells, the latter being virtually absent. The glandular lining epithelium is replaced by mucus-secreting goblet cells that resemble those lining the large intestine, a form of metaplasia referred to as intestinalisation. Some of the cells, as well as their nuclei, may increase to double the normal size, a form of 'megaloblastic' change exactly analogous to that seen in the marrow. As will be seen, patients with pernicious anaemia have a higher incidence of gastric cancer. The gastric atrophic and metaplastic changes are the result of autoimmunity and not vitamin B_{12} deficiency; hence, parenteral administration of vitamin B_{12} corrects the bone marrow changes, but gastric atrophy and achlorhydria persist.

Crohn's disease involving the stomach is quite uncommon. The inflammation with Crohn's disease is transmural. Linitis plastica characterises a diffuse cancer with a poor prognosis.

3.44

Answer: E

The term 'Hodgkin's lymphoma' (HL), previously known as Hodgkin's disease, encompasses a group of lymphoid neoplasms that differ

pathology

from non-Hodgkin's lymphoma (NHL) in several respects. Although NHL frequently occurs at extranodal sites and spreads in an unpredictable fashion, HL arises in a single node or chain of nodes and spreads first to the anatomically contiguous nodes. It is characterised morphologically by the presence of distinctive neoplastic giant cells called Reed–Sternberg cells, which induce the accumulation of reactive lymphocytes, histiocytes (macrophages) and granulocytes. Reed–Sternberg cells are multinucleated with large nucleoli. Variants called lacunar cells are also seen with some forms of Hodgkin's disease.

TB results in a characteristic granulomatous inflammatory reaction that forms both caseating and non-caseating tubercles. The granulomata are usually enclosed within a fibroblastic rim punctuated by lymphocytes. Multinucleate giant cells are present in the granulomata. A monomorphous proliferation of intermediate-sized lymphoid cells is seen with Burkitt's lymphoma, often with accompanying macrophages. Mycosis fungoides (despite the name) is not a fungal disease, but a form of cutaneous T-cell lymphoma. A proliferation of plasma cells leads to multiple myeloma, usually detected by monoclonal immunoglobulin production.

3.45

Answer: A

Seminomas are the most common type of germinal tumour (50%) and the type most likely to produce a uniform population of cells. They almost never occur in infants; they peak in those in their 30s. Seminomas produce bulky masses, sometimes ten times the size of the normal testis. The typical seminoma has a homogeneous, grey–white, lobulated, cut surface, usually devoid of haemorrhage or necrosis. In more than half of cases, the entire testis is replaced. Generally, the tunica albuginea is not penetrated, but occasionally, extension to the epididymis, spermatic cord or scrotal sac occurs. The tumour markers are not markedly elevated.

Choriocarcinomas are very aggressive tumours. A high hCG (human chorionic gonadotrophin) would suggest a component of choriocarcinoma. A high AFP (α-fetoprotein) would suggest embryonal carcinoma or yolk sac carcinoma. Embryonal carcinomas

pathology

occur mostly in the 20- to 30-year age group. These tumours are more aggressive than seminomas. The yolk sac tumour is also known as infantile embryonal carcinoma or endodermal sinus tumour; it is of interest because it is the most common testicular tumour in infants and children aged up to 3 years. In this age group, it has a very good prognosis. In adults, the pure form of this tumour is rare; instead, yolk sac elements frequently occur in combination with embryonal carcinoma. Tumours of Leydig cells are particularly interesting because they may produce androgens or combinations of androgens and oestrogens, and some have also produced corticosteroids. They arise at any age, although most of the reported cases have been noted between 20 and 60 years of age. As with other testicular tumours, the most common presenting feature is testicular swelling, but, in some patients, gynaecomastia may be the first symptom. In children, hormonal effects, manifested primarily as sexual precocity, are the dominating feature. About 10% of the tumours in adults are invasive and produce metastases; most are benign.

3.46

Answer: D

Cryptorchidism is synonymous with undescended testes and is found in about 1% of 1-year-old boys. This anomaly represents a complete or incomplete failure of the intra-abdominal testes to descend into the scrotal sac. It usually occurs as an isolated anomaly but may be accompanied by other malformations of the genitourinary tract, such as hypospadias. In this case the testis has been out of place too long to retain any function of spermatogenesis. It is now atrophic with few remaining germ cells and minimal, if any, spermatogenesis occurring. A cryptorchid testis at this age no longer functions and presents a risk for subsequent development of seminoma. The earlier in life that an orchidopexy is performed, generally under the age of 5, the more likely that the testis will function properly.

The opposite testis will not be affected by the cryptorchid testis. The patient still has one good testis. Even with bilateral cryptorchidism, the Leydig cells of the testicular interstitium continue to function and produce testosterone. If this were testicular feminisation with androgen insensitivity, the phenotype would be female. If he had Klinefelter syndrome, the testes would be small and in the scrotum.

pathology

3.47

Answer: E

A prostatic nodule at this age strongly suggests carcinoma. In about 70% of cases, carcinoma of the prostate arises in the peripheral zone of the gland, classically in a posterior location, often rendering it palpable on rectal examination. Microscopically, prostatic adenocarcinomas have irregular glands without intervening stroma. Large nucleoli are characteristic.

Hyperplasia is usually not a focal process, and the glands are not small and crowded. Inflammation is usually not focal in the prostate. The most common tumour to involve the prostate secondarily is urothelial cancer. Two distinct patterns of involvement exist. Large, invasive, urothelial cancers can directly invade from the bladder into the prostate. Alternatively, carcinoma *in situ* of the bladder can extend into the prostatic urethra and down into the prostatic ducts and acini. Metastatic urothelial carcinoma would be an unusual pattern of metastasis. Urothelial carcinomas do not appear glandular. The glands around an infarct may show squamous metaplasia, but they will not be small and crowded.

3.48

Answer: B

Exposure to the allergens of a bee sting is a cause for systemic anaphylaxis for some people. A bee sting will precipitate a type I hypersensitivity reaction and adrenaline (epinephrine) can be life saving in this situation.

Local immune complexes are a feature of type III hypersensitivity with farmer's lung. Macrophages have a major role with type IV hypersensitivity reactions. Myasthenia gravis is an example of an anti-receptor disease of an autoimmune nature (type II hypersensitivity). Antibody is directed against acetylcholine (ACh) receptors. Many myasthenia gravis patients have a thymoma or thymic hyperplasia. Complement activation is a feature of type III hypersensitivity reactions.

3.49

Answer: B

About 20% of nodules that are hypofunctioning (cold) on a thyroid scintiscan are malignant, but most are benign. Hyperfunctioning (hot) nodules carry a low risk of malignancy, but exceptions occur. Ultrasonography is a sensitive method for determining whether a lesion is solid or cystic, but it cannot distinguish between benign and malignant nodules. Although thyroid cysts have a lower likelihood of being malignant, larger carcinomas can undergo cystic degeneration. Excision biopsy in the form of total lobectomy on the affected side, with isthmusectomy preserving the recurrent laryngeal nerves and parathyroids, not only aids in getting rid of the thyroid nodule, especially in patients with cancer phobia, but also provides adequate tissue for definitive histopathological diagnosis. Fine-needle aspiration cytology (FNAC) is able to tell only whether a neoplasm is benign, malignant or indeterminate (suspicious). It can diagnose papillary carcinoma but mostly the actual type of a neoplasm cannot be determined by FNAC. Sudden increase in the size of a solitary nodule over a period of 24 h is usually the result of haemorrhage in a pre-existing nodule and not a sign of malignancy.

3.50

Answer: A

There is an enormous amount of experimental and epidemiological data to support the role of tamoxifen as a chemopreventive agent in breast cancer. Tamoxifen is the oldest of all the selective oestrogen receptor modulators. It is prescribed for women with hormone-receptor-positive breast cancer before and after menopause. Tamoxifen causes breast epithelial cells to rest in G0; it induces apoptosis in tumours; in the adjuvant setting it reduces the risk of contralateral breast cancers. It is likely that tamoxifen acts not only through its oestrogen-blocking activity but also through other mechanisms independent of oestrogen receptors (ERs), such as stimulation of tissue fibroblasts to produce the negative paracrine growth factor called TGF (transforming growth factor). Tamoxifen also reduces the circulating levels of insulin-like growth factor I, which not only is a mitogen for breast epithelium but also stimulates the motility and metastatic potential of malignant cells.

pathology

Tamoxifen also influences activities of two other important enzymes: protein kinase C and calmodulin-dependent cAMP phosphodiesterase. Recently, tamoxifen has been shown to inhibit angiogenesis and induce apoptosis. These other mechanisms of action of tamoxifen probably explain the counterintuitive response to tamoxifen seen among postmenopausal, ER-negative women in the world overview. Tamoxifen therapy is particularly effective in elderly postmenopausal women and is being used as the only initial treatment in this age group, with complete resolution of the tumours in 50% and reduction in size in a further 20%.

In a number of centres, patients aged 70 years and above are treated with tamoxifen (40 mg daily) and surgical treatment is considered only if there is no response to the initial treatment. In premenopausal patients, 5 years of adjuvant tamoxifen reduces the risk of recurrence and death, irrespective of whether chemotherapy has been given. Tamoxifen exerts a highly beneficial effect on bone metabolism, lipid profile and the myocardium. Tamoxifen reduces the risk of ischaemic heart disease by decreasing low-density lipoprotein (LDL)-cholesterol and osteoporosis by up to 50%. It has side-effects similar to those of natural oestrogens, including hot flushes, nausea, vomiting, skin rash, vaginal bleeding and discharge (resulting from some slight oestrogenic activity of the drug and some of its metabolites). Hypercalcaemia requiring cessation of the drug may occur. Tamoxifen can also lead to increased pain if the tumour has metastasised to bone. Tamoxifen has the potential to cause endometrial cancer.

3.51

Answer: E

Papillary thyroid carcinoma, comprising 85% of thyroid carcinomas, occurs in any age group but especially in children and women younger than 40. Classically it presents as a lump in the thyroid or less commonly as a solid swelling in a lymph node draining the thyroid, the primary in the thyroid being undetectable. Such a lymph node is often termed a 'lateral aberrant thyroid'. It has an excellent prognosis. The 5-year survival rate is 90%, which is scarcely reduced at 10 years. Involvement of cervical nodes does not affect the prognosis adversely. Papillary carcinoma may be multifocal and metastasises to cervical lymph nodes. Its treatment by total thyroidectomy with preservation of the parathyroids is one school of thought on treatment. Another school of thought feels that this is rather too radical for a disease carrying such an excellent outlook and advises total thyroid lobectomy on the affected side with subtotal lobectomy on the contralateral side. There is a third approach that advocates only local removal of the tumour and T3 suppression of TSH.

3.52

Answer: A

Vitamin K is a required cofactor for a liver microsomal carboxylase that is necessary to convert glutamyl residues in certain protein precursors to γ-carboxyglutamates. Clotting factors VII, IX and X, and prothrombin all require carboxylation of glutamate residues for functional activity. Carboxylation provides calcium-binding sites and thus allows calcium-dependent interaction of these clotting factors with a phospholipid surface involved in the generation of thrombin. In addition, activation of anticoagulant proteins C and S also requires glutamate carboxylation. In the course of the reaction of vitamin K with its substrate proteins, its active (reduced) form is oxidised to an epoxide but then it is promptly reduced back by a liver epoxide reductase. Thus, in a healthy liver, vitamin K is efficiently recycled, and the daily dietary requirement is low.

Furthermore, endogenous intestinal bacterial flora readily synthesise the vitamin. Deficiency usually occurs: (1) in fat malabsorption syndromes, particularly with biliary tract disease, as with the other fat-soluble vitamins; (2) after destruction of the endogenous vitamin K-synthesising flora, particularly with ingestion of broad-spectrum antibiotics; (3) in the neonatal period, when liver reserves are small, the bacterial flora not yet developed and the level of vitamin K in breast milk low; and (4) in diffuse liver disease, even in the presence of normal vitamin K stores, because hepatocyte dysfunction interferes with synthesis of the vitamin K-dependent coagulation factors. In patients with thromboembolic disease, therapeutically desirable vitamin K deficiency is induced by coumarin anticoagulants

pathology

(eg warfarin). These agents block the activity of liver epoxide reductase and thereby prevent regeneration of reduced vitamin K. The major consequence of vitamin K deficiency (or of inefficient use of vitamin K by the liver) is the development of a bleeding diathesis.

3.53

Answer: B

The ultimate step in the elimination of infectious agents and necrotic cells is their killing and degradation within neutrophils and macrophages, which occur most efficiently after activation of the phagocytes. Microbial killing is accomplished largely by oxygen-dependent mechanisms. Phagocytosis stimulates a burst in oxygen consumption, glycogenolysis, increased glucose oxidation via the hexose monophosphate shunt and production of reactive oxygen intermediates (ROIs, also called reactive oxygen species). The generation of ROIs is the result of the rapid activation of an oxidase (NADPH oxidase), which oxidises NADPH (reduced nicotinamide adenine dinucleotide phosphate) and, in the process, reduces oxygen to the superoxide anion. Superoxide is then converted into hydrogen peroxide (H_2O_2), mostly by spontaneous dismutation. Hydrogen peroxide can also be further reduced to the highly reactive hydroxyl radical. Most of the H_2O_2 is eventually broken down by catalase into H_2O and O_2, and some is destroyed by the action of glutathione oxidase.

NADPH oxidase is an enzyme complex consisting of at least seven proteins. In resting neutrophils, different NADPH oxidase protein components are located in the plasma membrane and the cytoplasm. In response to activating stimuli, the cytosolic protein components translocate to the plasma membrane or phagosomal membrane, where they assemble and form the functional enzyme complex. Thus, the ROIs are produced within the lysosome where the ingested substances are segregated, and the cell's own organelles are protected from the harmful effects of the ROIs. Defects in the NADPH oxidase system will affect the generation of ROIs. Bactericidal permeability, increasing protein, lysozyme, major basic proteins and defensins are all oxygen-independent mechanisms that help accomplish bacterial killing by leukocytes.

3.54

Answer: C

The complement system consists of 20 component proteins (and their cleavage products), which are found in their greatest concentration in the plasma. This system functions in both innate and adaptive immunity for defence against microbial agents. In the process of complement activation, a number of complement components are elaborated that cause increased vascular permeability, chemotaxis and opsonisation.

Complement proteins are present as inactive forms in plasma and are numbered C1–C9. Many of these proteins are activated to become proteolytic enzymes that degrade other complement proteins, thus forming a cascade capable of tremendous enzymatic amplification. The critical step in the elaboration of the biological functions of complement is the activation of the third (and most abundant) component: C3. Cleavage of C3 can occur by one of three pathways: the classic pathway, which is triggered by fixation of C1 to antibody (IgM or IgG) combined with antigen; the alternative pathway, which can be triggered by microbial surface molecules (eg endotoxin or lipopolysaccharide), complex polysaccharides, cobra venom and other substances, in the absence of antibody; and the lectin pathway, in which plasma mannose-binding lectin binds to carbohydrates on microbes and directly activates C1.

Whichever pathway is involved in the early steps of complement activation, they all lead to the formation of an active enzyme called the C3 convertase, which splits C3 into two functionally distinct fragments: C3a and C3b. C3a is released and C3b becomes covalently attached to the cell or molecule where complement is being activated. C3b then binds to the previously generated fragments to form C5 convertase, which cleaves C5 to release C5a. The remaining C5b binds the late components (C6–C9), culminating in the formation of the membrane attack complex (MAC, composed of multiple C9 molecules).

pathology

3.55

Answer: D

The kinin system generates vasoactive peptides from plasma proteins, called kininogens, by the action of specific proteases called kallikreins. Activation of the kinin system results in the release of the vasoactive nonapeptide bradykinin. Bradykinin increases vascular permeability and causes contraction of smooth muscle, dilatation of blood vessels and pain when injected into the skin. These effects are similar to those of histamine. The cascade that eventually produces kinins is triggered by activation of Hageman factor (factor XII of the intrinsic clotting pathway) on contact with negatively charged surfaces, such as collagen and basement membranes. A fragment of factor XII (prekallikrein activator or factor XIIa) is produced, and this converts plasma prekallikrein into an active proteolytic form, the enzyme kallikrein. The latter cleaves a plasma glycoprotein precursor, high-molecular-weight kininogen, to produce bradykinin. High-molecular-weight kininogen also acts as a cofactor or catalyst in the activation of Hageman factor. The action of bradykinin is short-lived because it is quickly inactivated by an enzyme called kininase. Any remaining kinin is inactivated during the passage of plasma through the lung by angiotensin-converting enzyme (ACE). Kallikrein itself is a potent activator of Hageman factor, allowing for autocatalytic amplification of the initial stimulus. Kallikrein has chemotactic activity and also directly converts C5 to the chemoattractant product C5a.

3.56

Answer: E

Carcinoma of the gallbladder is slightly more common in women and occurs most frequently in the seventh decade of life. Only rarely is it discovered at a resectable stage, and the mean 5-year survival rate has remained for many years at about 1%, despite surgical intervention. Gallstones are present in 60–90% of cases. In Asia, where pyogenic and parasitic diseases of the biliary tree are common, the coexistence of gallstones is much lower. Presumably, gallbladders containing stones or infectious agents develop cancer as a result of irritative trauma and chronic inflammation. Carcinogenic derivatives of bile acids may also play a role. Most carcinomas of the gallbladder are adenocarcinomas. Some are papillary in architecture and are well to moderately differentiated; others are infiltrative and poorly differentiated to undifferentiated. About 5% are squamous cell carcinomas or have adenosquamous differentiation. A minority may exhibit carcinoid or a variety of mesenchymal features. By the time these neoplasms are discovered, most have invaded the liver centrifugally, and many have extended to the cystic duct and adjacent bile ducts and portahepatic lymph nodes. The peritoneum, gastrointestinal tract and lungs are common sites of seeding.

3.57

Answer: C

The histology is characteristic of pleomorphic adenoma. These neoplasms have also been called mixed tumours. They represent about 60% of tumours in the parotid, are less common in the submandibular glands and are relatively rare in the minor salivary glands. They are benign tumours that are derived from a mixture of ductal (epithelial) and myoepithelial cells, and therefore they show both epithelial and mesenchymal differentiation. They also reveal epithelial elements dispersed throughout a matrix along with varying degrees of myxoid, hyaline, chondroid (cartilaginous) and even osseous tissue. In some tumours, the epithelial elements predominate; in others, they are present only in widely dispersed foci. Little is known about the origins of these neoplasms except that radiation exposure increases the risk. Equally uncertain is the histogenesis of the various components. A currently popular view is that all neoplastic elements, including those that appear to be mesenchymal, are of either myoepithelial or ductal reserve cell origin (hence the designation pleomorphic adenoma). Most pleomorphic adenomas present as rounded, well-demarcated masses rarely exceeding 6 cm in the greatest dimension. Although they are encapsulated, in some locations (particularly the palate) the capsule is not fully developed, and the expansile growth produces tongue-like protrusions into the surrounding gland, rendering enucleation of the tumour hazardous. The cut surface is grey–white with myxoid and blue translucent areas of chondroid.

pathology

3.58

Answer: B

The clinical picture in this case is suggestive of fat embolism. Fat embolism syndrome is characterised by pulmonary insufficiency, neurological symptoms, anaemia and thrombocytopenia. Microscopic fat globules may be found in the circulation after fractures of long bones (which have fatty marrow) or, rarely, in the setting of soft-tissue trauma and burns. Presumably the fat is released by marrow or adipose tissue injury and enters the circulation by rupture of marrow vascular sinusoids or venules. Although traumatic fat embolism occurs in some 90% of individuals with severe skeletal injuries, less than 10% of such patients have any clinical findings. Symptoms typically begin 1–3 days after injury, with sudden onset of tachypnoea, dyspnoea and tachycardia. Neurological symptoms include irritability and restlessness, with progression to delirium or coma. Patients may present with thrombocytopenia, presumably caused by platelets adhering to the myriad fat globules and being removed from the circulation; anaemia may result as a consequence of erythrocyte aggregation and haemolysis. A diffuse petechial rash in non-dependent areas (related to rapid onset of thrombocytopenia) is seen in 20–50% of cases and is useful in establishing a diagnosis. In its full-blown form, the syndrome is fatal in up to 10% of cases.

The pathogenesis of fat emboli syndrome probably involves both mechanical obstruction and biochemical injury. Microemboli of neutral fat cause occlusion of the pulmonary and cerebral microvasculature, aggravated by local platelet and erythrocyte aggregation; this is further exacerbated by release of free fatty acids from the fat globules, causing local toxic injury to endothelium. Platelet activation and recruitment of granulocytes (with free radical, protease and eicosanoid release) complete the vascular assault.

pathology

3.59

Answer: A

Primary mediators contained within mast-cell granules can be divided into three categories:

1. Biogenic amines: the most important vasoactive amine is histamine, which causes intense smooth muscle contraction, increased vascular permeability and increased secretion by nasal, bronchial and gastric glands.
2. Enzymes: these are contained in the granule matrix and include neutral proteases (chymase, tryptase) and several acid hydrolases. The enzymes cause tissue damage and lead to the generation of kinins and activated components of complement (eg C3a) by acting on their precursor proteins.
3. Proteoglycans: these include heparin, a well-known anticoagulant, and chondroitin sulphate. The proteoglycans serve to package and store the other mediators in the granules.

3.60

Answer: D

Fever, characterised by an elevation of body temperature, usually by 1–4°C, is one of the most prominent manifestations of the acute-phase response, especially when inflammation is associated with infection. Fever is produced in response to substances called pyrogens that act by stimulating prostaglandin synthesis in the vascular and perivascular cells of the hypothalamus. Bacterial products, such as lipopolysaccharides (called exogenous pyrogens), stimulate leukocytes to release cytokines such as IL-1 and TNF (called endogenous pyrogens), which increase the enzymes (cyclo-oxygenases) that convert arachidonic acid into prostaglandins. In the hypothalamus, the prostaglandins, especially PGE_2, stimulate the production of neurotransmitters such as cAMP, which function to reset the temperature set-point at a higher level. Non-steroidal anti-inflammatory drugs (NSAIDs), including aspirin, reduce fever by inhibiting cyclo-oxygenase and thus blocking prostaglandin synthesis.

pathology

3.61

Answer: E

Acute-phase proteins are plasma proteins, mostly synthesised in the liver, with plasma concentrations that may increase several hundredfold as part of the response to inflammatory stimuli. Three of the best-known examples of these proteins are C-reactive protein (CRP), fibrinogen and serum amyloid A (SAA). Synthesis of these molecules by hepatocytes is upregulated by cytokines, especially IL-6 (for CRP and fibrinogen) and IL-1 or TNF (for SAA). Many acute-phase proteins, such as CRP and SAA, bind to microbial cell walls, and may act as opsonins and fix complement. They also bind chromatin, possibly aiding in the clearing of necrotic cell nuclei. During the acute-phase response, SAA replaces apolipoprotein A, a component of high-density lipoprotein (HDL) particles. This may alter the targeting of HDLs from liver cells to macrophages, which can use these particles as a source of energy-producing lipids. The rise in fibrinogen causes erythrocytes to form stacks (rouleaux) that sediment more rapidly at unit gravity than individual erythrocytes. This is the basis for measuring the erythrocyte sedimentation rate (ESR) as a simple test for the systemic inflammatory response, caused by any number of stimuli, including lipopolysaccharides. Acute-phase proteins have beneficial effects during acute inflammation, but prolonged production of these proteins (especially SAA) causes secondary amyloidosis in chronic inflammation. Elevated serum levels of CRP are now used as a marker for increased risk of myocardial infarction in patients with coronary artery disease. It is believed that inflammation involving atherosclerotic plaques in the coronary arteries may predispose to thrombosis and subsequent infarction, and CRP is produced during inflammation.

3.62

Answer: A

Aldosterone is the main sodium-retaining hormone produced by the adrenal glands. It increases the reabsorption of sodium and water along with the excretion of potassium in the distal tubules of the kidneys. This action raises blood pressure. Hypoaldosteronism results in salt wasting, thereby decreasing serum sodium and increasing urine

pathology

sodium. As water follows sodium, the patient may develop orthostatic hypotension or become frankly hypotensive. In response to the electrical gradient established by sodium reabsorption, aldosterone induces the passive secretion of potassium at the distal convoluted tubule, promoting potassium excretion. Hypoaldosteronism would, in contrast, increase serum potassium and decrease urine potassium. Aldosterone causes hydrogen ions to be actively secreted into the distal tubule. Therefore, in hypoaldosteronism, H^+ ions are retained, creating a metabolic acidosis (decreased HCO_3^-).

3.63

Answer: B

This is a classical picture of cardiogenic shock. Cardiogenic shock is characterized by a decreased pumping ability of the heart that causes a shocklike state (ie global hypoperfusion). It most commonly occurs in association with, and as a direct result of, acute myocardial infarction. Similar to other shock states, cardiogenic shock is considered to be a clinical diagnosis characterized by decreased urine output, altered mentation, and hypotension. Other clinical characteristics include jugular venous distension, cardiac gallop, and pulmonary oedema. Cardiogenic shock is defined as sustained hypotension (systolic blood pressure less than 90 mmHg lasting more than 30 min) with evidence of tissue hypoperfusion with adequate left ventricular filling pressure. Tissue hypoperfusion is defined as cold peripheries (extremities colder than core), oliguria (< 30 ml/h), or both. In cardiogenic shock left ventricular function is compromised; therefore cardiac output is diminished. Preload is increased because blood from the right side of the heart and pulmonary circulation is pumped into an already filled left ventricle (this explains the S3 and S4 sounds). Pulmonary artery wedge pressure (PAWP) measured with a Swan–Ganz catheter, reveals left atrial pressure as well as left ventricular end-diastolic pressure and is elevated in heart failure. Increased left atrial pressure results in pulmonary oedema. Eventually, the right ventricle can no longer pump blood against the increased pulmonary pressure and fails. This causes a back up of blood which results in increased central venous pressure. Systemic vascular resistance is increased in an attempt to

pathology

compensate for diminished cardiac output. Mixed venous oxygen levels are reduced because of increased tissue demands for oxygen.

3.64

Answer: C

Acute tubular necrosis (ATN) is the death of tubular cells, which may result when tubular cells either do not get enough oxygen (ischaemic ATN) or have been exposed to a toxic drug or molecule (nephrotoxic ATN). Fortunately, new tubular cells usually replace those that have died. Indeed, the tubular cells of the kidneys undergo a continuous cycle of cell death and renewal, much like the cells of the skin. In the hospital setting, ATN is the most common cause of acute renal failure (ARF). Hospital patients often have acute medical problems that limit the oxygen supplied to the tubules or that cause tubular hypoperfusion (decreased blood flow).

Certain medical and surgical situations are associated with a high risk for developing ischaemic ATN:

- Hypotension (low blood pressure)
- Obstetric (birth-related) complications
- Obstructive jaundice (yellow-tinged skin caused by blocked flow of bile)
- Prolonged prerenal state
- Sepsis (infection in the blood or tissues)
- Surgery (eg open heart surgery, repair of abdominal aortic aneurysm).
  Some medications and clinical materials can cause nephrotoxic ATN:
  - aminoglycosides (antibacterial antibiotics such as streptomycin and gentamicin)
  - amphotericin B (antibiotic used to treat some forms of meningitis and systemic fungal infections)
  - cisplatin (anticancer agent used to treat late-stage ovarian and testicular cancers)
  - radioisotopic contrast media (agent used in certain imaging studies).

Exposure to certain molecules may also cause nephrotoxic ATN, eg when a person suffers significant muscle trauma, such as during a crush injury, the muscle enzyme creatine phosphokinase (CPK) leaks into the blood. Myoglobulin is the protein that leaks into the blood and ultimately causes ATN. Measurement of CPK is a marker of myoglobulin released by muscle cells. If enough CPK spills into the blood and is filtered through the glomeruli, it can damage the tubules, causing nephrotoxic ATN.

ATN typically does not produce specific signs or symptoms. Diagnosis is often supported by a positive history of risk factors. Yet the physician must rule out other reasons for ARF, such as prerenal, postrenal or renal ARF. Distinguishing ATN from prerenal ARF can be extremely difficult. Urine chemistry and microscopic examination of the urine help to confirm the diagnosis. ATN does not rapidly improve after the administration of large-volume intravenous fluid. Management relies on aggressive treatment of the factors that precipitated the ATN. One exception is the treatment of ATN associated with the breakdown of muscle fibres caused by a crush injury. Aggressive, forced diuresis (ie an increased excretion of urine) may improve the condition.

Patients at high risk for developing ARF from contrast-induced ATN should be treated with intravenous fluids before contrast exposure to prevent the ATN. There has been a recent report suggesting that pre-treatment of these patients with a medication called Mucomyst (acetylcysteine) may also help to prevent ARF in patients undergoing intravenous contrast exposure. As tubular cells have the capacity to replace themselves, the overall prognosis for ATN is quite good if the cause is corrected. Once the precipitating factor has been treated and removed, ATN usually resolves within 7–21 days. On occasion, the kidneys may not completely recover or (rarely) never recover, despite the resolution of other medical problems. This situation usually indicates that there is pre-existing, unidentified, renal dysfunction.

pathology

3.65

Answer: D

A ganglion cyst is a bump or mass that forms under the skin. A swelling on the back of the wrist or fingers is the most obvious sign. These cysts can be painless but are often associated with tenderness, which may restrict the range of movements. Most commonly, ganglia are seen on the wrist (usually the back side) and fingers, but they can also develop on the shoulder, elbow and knee. They form when tissues surrounding certain joints become inflamed and swell up with lubricating fluid, and can increase in size when the tissue is irritated or just appear to grow. However, they are not tumours or cancerous. Ganglia are harmless and if there is no pain or other complications they are usually left alone. They sometimes just disappear anyway.

Initial treatment may simply involve limiting the activities that place a strain on the affected area, resting the joint and supporting it in a splint. Draining the fluid from the cyst may help ease symptoms. If the ganglion is persistent surgical removal may be recommended. Ganglion cysts characteristically lack a true lining, which distinguishes them morphologically from synovial cysts.

3.66

Answer: D

This patient has Hodgkin's lymphoma (as suggested by the characteristic Reed–Sternberg cells). The most common presenting symptom for Hodgkin's lymphoma is painless lymph node enlargement, most frequently involving nodes on the neck. More generalised lymph node enlargement is also common, but systemic spread to the liver, lungs, bone narrow and other organs is usually a late event. Although localised disease usually occurs in lymph nodes above the diaphragm, isolated infradiaphragmatic disease may occur, and tends to be more common with the lymphocyte predominant type. Characteristic systemic symptoms, known as 'B' symptoms, are unexplained fevers, drenching night sweats and weight loss of > 10% of total body weight. Presence of these symptoms is an adverse prognostic factor. Other characteristic symptoms, although less clearly associated with poor prognosis, are fatigue, generalised pruritus and alcohol-induced pain in affected lymph nodes. The lymphatic spread of Hodgkin's lymphoma usually occurs in a stepwise fashion to contiguous lymph nodes. Anatomical staging, based on the Ann Arbor system (as shown below), has largely determined treatment decisions. The suffix 'B' is added to the stage category for patients with systemic symptoms (ie fever, night sweats and weight loss), whereas patients without systemic symptoms are designated 'A'.

Ann Arbor staging for Hodgkin's lymphoma

Stage	Description
I	Disease in single lymph node region
II	Disease in two or more regions on the same side of the diapragm
III	Disease in lymph node regions on both sides of the diaphragm
IV	Diffuse or disseminated disease in extralymphatic sites (eg liver and bone marrow) with or without lymph node involvement

The patient in this question has stage IIB disease because he has disease in two or more regions on the same side of the diapragm along with systemic symptoms.

3.67

Answer: E

This patient has symptoms suggestive of thoracic outlet obstruction caused by a cervical rib. Cervical ribs are an anomaly arising from the lowest cervical vertebrae but their relationship to the thoracic outlet syndrome is not such that the two conditions should be seen as synonymous. Perhaps no more than 10% of people who have cervical ribs develop the thoracic outlet syndrome and the syndrome may well occur in the absence of ribs. One problem in terms of diagnosis is that there may be a fibrous band that acts like a rib; however, not being calcified it does not appear on radiographs. There is also considerable controversy in the literature as to whether the condition actually

pathology

exists. Some authors claim that it is under-diagnosed whereas others say that it is over-diagnosed.

The syndrome involves compression, injury or irritation to the neurovascular structures at the root of the neck or upper thorax. The boundaries are the anterior and middle scalenes, the clavicle and first rib, with possible hypertrophy of the subclavius or under the pectoralis minor muscle. Compression may involve nerves, including the brachial plexus, usually the lower trunk or medial cord. It could involve compression of the subclavian artery, vein or both. Thrombosis, embolism or aneurysm of these vessels is less likely. With so much uncertainty and dispute over the diagnosis, it is not possible to give a meaningful figure for incidence but the true neurological type probably affects no more than one in a million. The overall incidence is given as between 3 and 80 per 1000. Onset is from the second to eighth decades with a peak in the fourth decade. It is more common in women than in men with an excess of between three- and ninefold.

3.68

Answer: A

Deficiency of iron is probably the most common nutritional disorder in the world. Although the prevalence of iron-deficiency anaemia is higher in developing countries, this form of anaemia is also common in the west, particularly in toddlers, adolescent girls and women of childbearing age. An iron deficiency can result from: (1) dietary lack, (2) impaired absorption, (3) increased requirement or (4) chronic blood loss. The dominating signs and symptoms frequently relate to the underlying cause of the anaemia, eg gastrointestinal or gynaecological disease, malnutrition, pregnancy and malabsorption.

The diagnosis of iron-deficiency anaemia ultimately rests on laboratory studies. Both the haemoglobin and haematocrit are depressed, usually to moderate levels, in association with hypochromia, microcytosis and some poikilocytosis. The serum iron and ferritin are low, and the total plasma iron-binding capacity (reflecting transferrin concentration) is high. Low serum iron with increased iron-binding capacity results in a reduction of transferrin saturation levels to below 15%. Reduced iron stores inhibit hepcidin synthesis and its serum levels fall. The level of soluble transferrin receptors, which are mostly derived from erythroid progenitors in the marrow, is elevated in iron deficiency as a result of a mild expansion of erythroid progenitors and an increased rate of transferrin receptor shedding. Reduced haem synthesis leads to elevation of free erythrocyte protoporphyrin. An alert clinician investigating unexplained iron-deficiency anaemia will occasionally discover an occult bleed or cancer and thereby save a life.

3.69

Answer: E

Vancomycin is the antibiotic of choice in this situation. Vancomycin is a parenteral glycopeptide antibiotic obtained from *Nocardia orientalis*. It is bactericidal and appears to exert its effect by binding to the precursor units of bacterial cell walls, inhibiting their synthesis. This binding occurs at a different site of action from that of penicillin. The net result is an alteration of bacterial cell wall permeability. In addition, RNA synthesis is inhibited. Perhaps as a result of this dual mechanism of action, resistance to vancomycin is uncommon, although it has been reported in strains of group D streptococci. Gram-negative organisms are not sensitive to vancomycin, perhaps because porin channels in the cell wall of the Gram-negative organism do not accommodate the large, bulky vancomycin molecule. Susceptible organisms are usually sensitive to concentrations of 1–5 μg/ml, even methicillin-resistant strains. It is effective for the treatment of Gram-positive infection caused by susceptible organism(s), particularly, staphylococcal infection including methicillin-sensitive *Staphylococcus aureus* (MSSA) and methicillin-resistant *Staphylococcus aureus* (MRSA), and for streptococcal and enterococcal infections in patients who are allergic to penicillin and other β-lactam antibiotics, in the following infections: endocarditis, bone and joint infections (eg osteomyelitis), lower respiratory tract infections (eg pneumonia), intra-abdominal infections (eg peritonitis), skin and skin structure infections (eg diabetic foot ulcer), bacteraemia or septicaemia, and urinary tract infection (UTI). In the average-sized adult, an initial dosage of 1000 mg i.v. or 15 mg/kg i.v. every 12 hours can be used, although individualisation of the dosage regimen may be necessary.

pathology

3.70

Answer: D

Aminoglycoside antibiotics such as streptomycin and gentamicin are commonly used throughout the world because of their low costs, high effectiveness and low rate of true resistance. They are active against a wide range of Gram-negative bacteria, as well as against *Staphylococcus aureus*, *Pseudomonas aeruginosa* and *Mycobacterium tuberculosis*. Aminoglycosides are used primarily for the treatment of life-threatening infections such as peritonitis, bacteraemia, pneumonia and endocarditis, as well as UTIs, cystic fibrosis and TB. However, their use is severely hampered by the risk of serious side-effects such as nephrotoxicity and ototoxicity, leading to kidney failure and hearing loss. Accumulation of aminoglycosides in vestibular and cochlear sensory cells of the inner ear leads to cell death, resulting in progressive hearing loss and vestibular dysfunction.

In contrast to aminoglycoside-mediated nephrotoxicity, effects on the cochlear and vestibular systems are largely irreversible. The effects are therefore cumulative with multiple rounds of treatment. The incidence of ototoxicity varies greatly, depending on the treatment regimen and the drugs used, ranging from 10–20% in the acute setting to up to 80% in patients receiving chronic therapy for TB. Deafness affects around 0.5–8% of treated individuals. Vestibular toxicity affects around 3%.

3.71

Answer: B

After exposure to hepatitis B virus (HBV), the long asymptomatic 4- to 26-week incubation period (mean: 6–8 weeks) is followed by acute disease lasting many weeks to months. Most patients experience a self-limited illness:

- HBsAg appears before the onset of symptoms, peaks during overt disease and then declines to undetectable levels in 3–6 months.

pathology

- HBeAg, HBV-DNA and DNA polymerase appear in the serum soon after HBsAg, and all signify active viral replication.
- IgM anti-HBc becomes detectable in serum shortly before the onset of symptoms, concurrent with the onset of elevation of serum aminotransferases. Over months, the IgM antibody is replaced by IgG anti-HBc.
- Anti-HBe is detectable shortly after the disappearance of HBeAg, implying that the acute infection has peaked and the disease is on the wane.
- IgG anti-HBs does not rise until the acute disease is over and is usually not detectable for a few weeks to several months after the disappearance of HBsAg. Anti-HBs may persist for life, conferring protection; this is the basis for current immunisation strategies using non-infectious HBsAg.

3.72

Answer: B

A variety of diseases has been found to be associated with certain HLA (human leukocyte antigen) alleles. The best known is the association between ankylosing spondylitis and HLA-B27; individuals who inherit this allele have a 90-fold greater chance (relative risk) of developing the disease than those who are negative for HLA-B27. The diseases that show association with the HLA locus can be broadly grouped into the following categories:

- Inflammatory diseases, including ankylosing spondylitis and several postinfectious arthropathies such as postgonococcal arthritis, all associated with HLA-B27
- Inherited errors of metabolism, such as 21-hydroxylase deficiency (HLA-BW47) and hereditary haemochromatosis (HLA-A)
- Autoimmune diseases, including autoimmune endocrinopathies, associated mainly with alleles at the DR locus.

pathology

295

3.73

Answer: C

Renal cell carcinomas represent about 1–3% of all visceral cancers and account for 85% of renal cancers in adults. The tumours occur most often in older individuals, usually in the sixth and seventh decades of life, showing a male preponderance in the ratio 2–3:1. As a result of their gross yellow colour and the resemblance of the tumour cells to clear cells of the adrenal cortex, they were at one time called hypernephromas. Tobacco is the most significant risk factor. Cigarette smokers have double the incidence of renal cell carcinoma of non-smokers, and pipe and cigar smokers are also more susceptible. The three classic diagnostic features of renal cell carcinoma are costovertebral pain, palpable mass and haematuria, but these are seen in only 10% of cases. The most reliable of the three is haematuria, but it is usually intermittent and may be microscopic; thus, the tumour may remain silent until it attains a large size. At this time, it gives rise to generalised constitutional symptoms, such as fever, malaise, weakness and weight loss. This pattern of asymptomatic growth occurs in many patients, so the tumour may have reached a diameter of more than 10 cm when it is discovered. In current times, however, many of these tumours are being discovered in the asymptomatic state by incidental radiological studies (eg CT or magnetic resonance imaging [MRI]) usually performed for non-renal indications.

Renal cell carcinoma is classified as one of the great mimics in medicine because it tends to produce a diversity of systemic symptoms not related to the kidney. In addition to the fever and constitutional symptoms mentioned earlier, renal cell carcinomas produce a number of paraneoplastic syndromes, ascribed to abnormal hormone production, including polycythaemia, hypercalcaemia, hypertension, hepatic dysfunction, feminisation or masculinisation, Cushing's syndrome, eosinophilia, leukaemoid reactions and amyloidosis. One of the common characteristics of this tumour is its tendency to metastasise widely before giving rise to any local symptoms or signs. In 25% of new patients with renal cell carcinoma, there is radiological evidence of metastases at the time of presentation. The most common locations of metastasis are the lungs (> 50%) and bones (33%), followed in order by the regional lymph nodes, liver and adrenals, and brain.

3.74

Answer: D

The measurement of serum thyroid-stimulating hormone (TSH) concentration using sensitive TSH (sTSH) assays provides the most useful single screening test for hyperthyroidism, because its levels are decreased even at the earliest stages, when the disease may still be subclinical. A low TSH value is usually confirmed with measurement of free T_4, which is expectedly increased. In an occasional patient, hyperthyroidism results predominantly from increased circulating levels of triiodothyronine (T_3; 'T_3 toxicosis'). In these cases, free T_4 levels may be decreased, and direct measurement of serum T_3 may be useful. In rare cases of pituitary-associated (secondary) hyperthyroidism, TSH levels are either normal or raised. Determining TSH levels after the injection of thyroid hormone-releasing hormone (TRH; TRH stimulation test) is used in the evaluation of cases of suspected hyperthyroidism with equivocal changes in the baseline serum TSH level. A normal rise in TSH after administration of TRH excludes secondary hyperthyroidism. Once the diagnosis of thyrotoxicosis has been confirmed by a combination of sTSH assays and free thyroid hormone levels, measurement of radioactive iodine uptake by the thyroid gland may be valuable in determining the aetiology, eg there may be diffusely increased uptake in the whole gland (Graves' disease), increased uptake in a solitary nodule (toxic adenoma) or decreased uptake (thyroiditis).

3.75

Answer: E

The proteins that apply brakes to cell proliferation are the products of tumour-suppressor genes. In a sense, the term 'tumour-suppressor genes' is a misnomer because the physiological function of these genes is to regulate cell growth, not to prevent tumour formation. As the loss of function of these genes is a key event in many, possibly all, human tumours and because their discovery resulted from the study of tumours, the name tumour suppressor persists. The *p53* tumour-suppressor gene is located on chromosome 17p13.1, and it is the most common target for genetic alteration in human tumours. A little over 50% of human tumours contain mutations in this gene. Homozygous

pathology

loss of *p53* gene activity can occur in virtually every type of cancer, including carcinomas of the lung, colon and breast – the three leading causes of cancer death. In most cases, the inactivating mutations affect both *p53* alleles and are acquired in somatic cells (not inherited in the germline). *S/S*, *INT–2*, *HST–1* and *HGF* are all proto-oncogenes.

3.76

Answer: A

Metabolic alkalosis is a primary increase in serum bicarbonate (HCO_3^-) concentration. This occurs as a consequence of a loss of H^+ from the body or a gain in HCO_3^-. In its pure form, it manifests as alkalaemia (pH > 7.40). As a compensatory mechanism, metabolic alkalosis leads to alveolar hypoventilation with a rise in arterial carbon dioxide tension ($Paco_2$), which diminishes the change in pH that would otherwise occur. The most common causes of metabolic alkalosis are the use of diuretics and the external loss of gastric secretions. Causes of metabolic alkalosis can be divided into chloride-responsive alkalosis (urine chloride < 20 mmol/l), chloride-resistant alkalosis (urine chloride > 20 mmol/l) and other causes, including alkali-loading alkalosis.

Loss of gastric secretions causes chloride-responsive alkalosis. Gastric secretions are rich in HCl. The secretion of HCl by the stomach usually stimulates bicarbonate secretion by the pancreas once HCl reaches the duodenum. Ordinarily, these substances are neutralised, and no net gain or loss of H^+ or HCO_3^- occurs. When HCl is lost by vomiting or nasogastric suction, pancreatic secretions are not stimulated and a net gain of HCO_3^- into the systemic circulation occurs, generating a metabolic alkalosis. Volume depletion maintains alkalosis. In this case, the hypokalaemia is secondary to the alkalosis itself and to renal loss of K^+ from the stimulation of aldosterone secretion. All other conditions in this question cause chloride-resistant alkalosis (urine chloride > 20 mmol/l).

3.77

Answer: B

Approximately 70–80% of patients with newly diagnosed bladder cancer will present with superficial bladder tumours (ie stage Ta, Tis or T1). Those who do present with superficial, non-invasive, bladder cancer can often be cured, and those with deeply invasive disease can sometimes be cured by surgery, irradiation or a combination of modalities that include chemotherapy. The clinical staging of carcinoma of the bladder is determined by the depth of invasion of the bladder wall by the tumour. This determination requires a cystoscopic examination, which includes a biopsy, and examination under anaesthesia to assess the size and mobility of palpable masses, the degree of induration of the bladder wall, and the presence of extravesical extension or invasion of adjacent organs. Clinical staging, even when CT and/or MRI and other imaging modalities are used, often underestimates the extent of the tumour, particularly in cancers that are less differentiated and more deeply invasive.

The American Joint Committee on Cancer (AJCC) has designated staging by TNM classification to define bladder cancer, as follows.

Primary tumour (T)

T_x: primary tumour cannot be assessed

T_0: no evidence of primary tumour

T_a: non-invasive papillary carcinoma

T_{IS}: carcinoma in situ (ie flat tumour)

T_1: tumour invades subepithelial connective tissue

T_2: tumour invades muscle

pT_{2a}: tumour invades superficial muscle (inner half)

pT_{2b}: tumour invades deep muscle (outer half)

T_3: tumour invades perivesical tissue

pT_{3a}: microscopically

pT_{3b}: macroscopically (extravesical mass)

pathology

T_4: tumour invades any of the following: prostate, uterus, vagina, pelvic wall or abdominal wall

T_{4a}: tumour invades the prostate, uterus, vagina

T_{4b}: tumour invades the pelvic wall, abdominal wall

The suffix 'm' should be added to the appropriate T category to indicate multiple lesions. The suffix 'IS' may be added to any T to indicate the presence of associated carcinoma in situ.

Regional lymph nodes (N)

N_x: regional lymph nodes cannot be assessed

N_0: no regional lymph node metastasis

N_1: metastasis in a single lymph node, $\leq$ 2 cm in greatest dimension

N_2: metastasis in a single lymph node, > 2 cm but $\leq$ 5 cm in greatest dimension; or multiple lymph nodes, $\leq$ 5 cm in greatest dimension

N_3: metastasis in a lymph node, > 5 cm in greatest dimension

Distant metastasis (M)

MX: Distant metastasis cannot be assessed

M0: No distant metastasis

M1: Distant metastasis

AJCC stage groupings

Stage 0a:	T_a, N_0, M_0
Stage 0_{IS}:	T_{IS}, N_0, M_0
Stage I:	T_1, N_0, M_0
Stage II:	T_{2a}, N_0, M_0
	T_{2b}, N_0, M_0
Stage III	T_{3a}, N_0, M_0
	T_{3b}, N_0, M_0
	T_{4a}, N_0, M_0

Stage IV T_{4b}, N_0, M_0

Any T, N_1, M_0

Any T, N_2, M_0

Any T, N_3, M_0

Any T, any N, M_1

Thus the patient in this question has stage II disease.

3.78

Answer: C

The patient in this question has ulcerative colitis as suggested by the bloody diarrhoea, rectal involvement and, especially, the continuous nature of the mucosal damage. In the list of options, pseudopolyps are the only feature that is characteristic of ulcerative colitis. All the other choices are features of Crohn's disease. The table below provides a comparison of ulcerative colitis and Crohn's disease.

Comparison of ulcerative colitis and Crohn's disease

Feature	Ulcerative colitis	Crohn's disease
Affected age group	Young to middle age	Young
Gross bleeding	Common	Common
Fistulae	Rare	Common
Thickened mesentery	Rare	Common
Enlarged mesenteric nodes	Rare	Common
Shortening of the colon	Common	Rare
Small bowel involvement	Never	Common
Thickening of the intestinal wall	Rare	Common
Strictures	Never	Common
Perforation	Common	Rare
Segmented effect	Never	Common
Pseudopolyps	Common	Rare

3.79

Answer: D

Acute pancreatitis causes the release of many digestive enzyme precursors, which are then converted to the active form in the damaged tissues. These enzymes degrade the adipose tissue around the pancreatic lobules, producing enzymatic fat necrosis. As part of this process, many free fatty acids are produced that can bind as soaps to extracellular calcium in chemical equilibrium with serum calcium. This often causes a significant decrease in serum calcium levels.

3.80

Answer: E

From a clinical standpoint, tumours of the testis are segregated into two broad categories: seminoma and non-seminomatous germ-cell tumours (NSGCTs). NSGCT is an umbrella designation that includes tumours of one histological type, such as embryonal cell carcinoma, as well as those with more than one histological pattern. NSGCTs behave differently from seminoma. Seminomas tend to remain localised to the testis for a long time; hence, about 70% present in clinical stage I. In contrast, about 60% of patients with NSGCTs present with advanced clinical disease (stages II and III). Metastases from seminomas typically involve lymph nodes. Haematogenous spread occurs later in the course of dissemination. NSGCTs not only metastasise earlier but also use the haematogenous route more frequently. The rare pure choriocarcinoma is the most aggressive of the NSGCTs. It might not cause any testicular enlargement but instead spreads predominantly and rapidly via the bloodstream. Therefore, the lungs and liver are involved early in virtually every case. From a therapeutic viewpoint, seminomas are extremely radiosensitive, whereas NSGCTs are relatively radioresistant. To summarise, compared with seminomas, NSGCTs are biologically more aggressive and in general have a poorer prognosis.

pathology

3.81

Answer: C

The most important prognostic indicator in lung cancer is the extent of disease. The Union Internationale Contre le Cancer (UICC) and the AJCC have developed the tumour, node and metastases (TNM) staging system, which takes into account the degree of spread of the primary tumour, the extent of regional lymph node involvement and the presence or absence of distant metastases. Non-small-cell lung cancer (NSCLC) accounts for about 75% of all lung cancers. NSCLC is subdivided into adenocarcinoma, squamous cell carcinoma and large cell carcinoma. Despite their histological and clinical differences, they share a similar prognosis and management and are staged by using the same TNM system. The TNM staging system takes into account: the degree of spread of the primary tumour, represented by T; the extent of regional lymph node involvement, represented by N; and the presence or absence of distant metastases, represented by M. The TNM system is used for all lung carcinomas except small cell lung cancers, which are staged separately. In the TNM systems, the tumour (T) stages are as follows:

- T_{IS}: carcinoma *in situ*
- T_x: positive malignant cytological findings, no lesion observed
- T_1: diameter ≤ 3 cm and surrounded by lung or visceral pleura or endobronchial tumour distal to the lobar bronchus
- T_2: diameter > 3 cm; extension to the visceral pleura, atelectasis or obstructive pneumopathy involving less than one lung; lobar endobronchial tumour; or tumour of a main bronchus > 2 cm from the carina
- T_3: tumour at the apex; total atelectasis of one lung; endobronchial tumour of main bronchus within 2 cm of the carina but not invading it; or tumour of any size with direct extension to the adjacent structures such as the chest wall, mediastinal pleura, diaphragm, pericardium parietal layer or mediastinal fat of the phrenic nerve
- T_4: invasion of the mediastinal organs, including the oesophagus, trachea, carina, great vessels and/or heart; obstruction of the superior vena cava; involvement of a

pathology

vertebral body; recurrent nerve involvement; malignant
pleural or pericardial effusion; or satellite pulmonary
nodules within the same lobe as the primary tumour.

Thus, according to TNM staging the patient in this question has a T_2
tumour.

3.82

Answer: B

This patient has Buerger's disease, also known as thromboangiitis
obliterans. It is a distinctive disease that often leads to vascular
insufficiency. It is characterised by segmental, thrombosing, acute
and chronic inflammation of medium-sized and small arteries,
principally the tibial and radial arteries and sometimes secondarily
extending to the veins and nerves of the extremities. Previously a
condition that occurred almost exclusively among heavy cigarette-
smoking men, Buerger's disease has been increasingly reported in
women, probably reflecting smoking increases among women. The
disease begins before age 35 in most cases. Later complications are
chronic ulcerations of the toes, feet or fingers, and frank gangrene in
some patients. In contrast to atherosclerosis, Buerger's disease
involves smaller arteries and is accompanied by severe pain, even at
rest, related undoubtedly to the neural involvement. Abstinence from
cigarette smoking in the early stages of the disease often prevents
further attacks.

Wegener's granulomatosis is a necrotising vasculitis characterised by
the triad of: (1) acute necrotising granulomata of the upper
respiratory tract (ear, nose, sinuses, throat), lower respiratory tract
(lung) or both; (2) necrotising or granulomatous vasculitis affecting
small to medium-sized vessels (eg capillaries, venules, arterioles and
arteries), most prominent in the lungs and upper airways but
affecting other sites as well; and (3) renal disease in the form of focal
necrotising, often crescentic, glomerulitis.

Kawasaki's disease is an arteritis that often involves the coronary
arteries, usually in young children and infants (80% of cases are
younger than 4), and is the leading cause of acquired heart disease in
children in North America and Japan. It is associated with the

mucocutaneous lymph node syndrome, an acute but usually self-limited illness manifested by fever, conjunctival and oral erythema and erosion, oedema of the hands and feet, erythema of the palms and soles, a skin rash often with desquamation and enlargement of cervical lymph nodes.

Polyarteritis nodosa is a systemic vasculitis of small or medium-sized muscular arteries (but not arterioles, capillaries or venules), typically involving renal and visceral vessels but sparing the pulmonary circulation. Clinical manifestations result from ischaemia and infarction of affected tissues and organs.

Takayasu's arteritis is a granulomatous vasculitis of medium and larger arteries; described in 1908 by Takayasu, it is characterised principally by ocular disturbances and marked weakening of the pulses in the upper extremities (pulseless disease). The pathological findings that account for the clinical picture are vasculitis and subsequent fibrous thickening of the aorta, particularly the aortic arch and its branches, with narrowing or virtual obliteration of the origins or more distal portions. The illness is seen predominantly in women aged under 40. The cause and pathogenesis are unknown, although autoimmune mechanisms are suspected. A high frequency of the HLA haplotype A24-B52-DR2 has been found in Japanese patients but not in other populations.

3.83

Answer: A

Peutz–Jeghers syndrome is a rare autosomal dominant syndrome characterised by multiple hamartomatous polyps scattered throughout the entire gastrointestinal tract and melanotic mucosal, and cutaneous pigmentation around the lips, oral mucosa, face, genitalia and palmar surfaces of the hands. Patients with this syndrome are at risk for intussusception, which is a common cause of mortality. The Peutz–Jeghers polyps tend to be large and pedunculated with a firm lobulated contour. The distribution of polyps in patients is reported as follows: stomach 25%; colon 30%; and small bowel 100%. Although these hamartomatous polyps themselves do not have malignant potential, patients with the syndrome have an increased risk of developing carcinomas of the

pathology

pancreas, breast, lung, ovary and uterus. The well-documented and characteristic tumours include sex cord tumours of the ovary, adenoma malignum of the uterine cervix and Sertoli cell tumours of the testis. When gastrointestinal adenocarcinoma occurs, it arises from concomitant adenomatous lesions. The underlying genetic basis for the Peutz–Jeghers syndrome is the mutation of gene *STK11* (*LKB1*) located on chromosome 19. The gene encodes a protein with serine/threonine kinase activity.

All other syndromes are characterised by adenomatous polyps.

3.84

Answer: E

The seronegative spondyloarthropathies are a group of diseases that develop in genetically predisposed individuals and are initiated by environmental factors, especially prior infections or exposures. The manifestations are immune mediated and may be triggered by a T-cell response to unknown antigens. Clinically, the diseases produce inflammatory peripheral or axial arthritis and inflammation of tendinous attachments. The seronegative spondyloarthropathies include ankylosing spondylitis, reactive arthritis (Reiter's syndrome and enteritis-associated arthritis), psoriatic arthritis and arthritis associated with inflammatory bowel disease (ulcerative colitis, Crohn's disease). They share overlapping clinical features, and many are associated with HLA-B27 and a triggering infection.

3.85

Answer: B

Secondary mediators include two classes of compounds: lipid mediators and cytokines. The lipid mediators are generated by sequential reactions in the mast-cell membranes that lead to activation of phospholipase A_2, an enzyme that acts on membrane phospholipids to yield arachidonic acid. This is the parent compound from which leukotrienes and prostaglandins are derived by the 5-lipoxygenase and cyclo-oxygenase pathways.

- Leukotrienes: leukotrienes LTC_4 and LTD_4 are the most potent vasoactive and spasmogenic agents known. On a molar basis, they are several thousand times more active than histamine in increasing vascular permeability and causing bronchial smooth muscle contraction. LTB_4 is highly chemotactic for neutrophils, eosinophils and monocytes.
- Prostaglandin D_2: this is the most abundant mediator derived by the cyclo-oxygenase pathway in mast cells. It causes intense bronchospasm as well as increased mucus secretion.
- Platelet-activating factor (PAF): PAF is produced by some mast-cell populations. It causes platelet aggregation, release of histamine, bronchospasm, increased vascular permeability and vasodilatation. In addition, it has important pro-inflammatory actions. PAF is chemotactic for neutrophils and eosinophils. At high concentrations, it activates the newly recruited inflammatory cells, causing them to aggregate and degranulate. As a result of its ability to recruit and activate inflammatory cells, it is considered important in the initiation of the late-phase response. Although the production of PAF is also triggered by the activation of phospholipase A_2, it is not a product of arachidonic acid metabolism.
- Cytokines: mast cells are sources of many cytokines, which play an important role in the late-phase reaction of immediate hypersensitivity because of their ability to recruit and activate inflammatory cells. The cytokines include TNF, IL-1, IL-3, IL-4, IL-5, IL-6 and GM-CSF (granulocyte–macrophage colony-stimulating factor), as well as chemokines, such as macrophage inflammatory protein (MIP)-1a and MIP-1β. Mast cell-derived TNF and chemokines are important mediators of the inflammatory response seen at the site of allergic inflammation. Inflammatory cells that accumulate at the sites of type I hypersensitivity reactions are additional sources of cytokines and histamine-releasing factors that cause further mast-cell degranulation.

pathology

3.86

Answer: A

Carcinoid tumour is derived from resident endocrine cells, with the gastrointestinal tract and lung as the predominant sites of occurrence. The peak incidence of these neoplasms is in the sixth decade, but they may appear at any age. They comprise less than 2% of colorectal malignancies but almost half of small intestinal malignant tumours. The appendix is the most common site of gut carcinoid tumours, followed by the small intestine (primarily ileum), rectum, stomach and colon. However, the rectal tumours may represent up to half of tumours that come to clinical attention. Those that arise in the stomach and ileum are frequently multicentric, but the remainder tend to be solitary lesions. In the appendix they appear as bulbous swellings of the tip, which frequently obliterate the lumen. Elsewhere in the gut, they appear as intramural or submucosal masses that create small, polypoid or plateau-like elevations rarely > 3 cm in diameter.

Gastrointestinal carcinoids only rarely produce local symptoms, which are caused by angulation or obstruction of the small intestine. Many (especially rectal and appendiceal) are asymptomatic and found incidentally. Appendiceal and rectal carcinoids infrequently metastasise, even though they may show extensive local spread. By contrast, 90% of ileal, gastric and colonic carcinoids that have penetrated halfway through the muscle wall have spread to lymph nodes and distant sites such as the liver at the time of diagnosis. This is especially true for tumours > 2 cm in diameter. Carcinoid syndrome occurs in about 1% of all patients with carcinoids and in 20% of those with widespread metastases. The overall 5-year survival rate for carcinoids (excluding appendiceal) is about 90%. Even with small-bowel tumours with hepatic metastases, it is better than 50%. However, widespread disease will usually cause death.

3.87

Answer: C

Up to 40% of lymphomas arise in sites other than lymph nodes, and the gut is the most common location. Conversely, about 1–4% of all gastrointestinal malignancies are lymphomas. By definition, primary gastrointestinal lymphomas exhibit no evidence of liver, spleen, mediastinal lymph node or bone marrow involvement at the time of diagnosis – regional lymph node involvement may be present. Primary gastrointestinal lymphomas usually arise as sporadic neoplasms but also occur more frequently in certain patient populations:

- Chronic gastritis caused by *Helicobacter pylori*
- Chronic sprue-like syndromes
- Natives of the Mediterranean region
- Congenital immunodeficiency states
- Infection with HIV
- After organ transplantation with immunosuppression.

3.88

Answer: B

The clinical features and laboratory investigations are suggestive of Addison's disease. Addison's disease begins insidiously and does not come to attention until at least 90% of the cortex of both glands is destroyed and the levels of circulating glucocorticoids and mineralocorticoids are significantly decreased. The initial manifestations include progressive weakness and easy fatiguability, which may be dismissed as non-specific complaints.

Gastrointestinal disturbances are common and include anorexia, nausea, vomiting, weight loss and diarrhoea. In patients with primary adrenal disease, increased circulating levels of the ACTH precursor hormone stimulate melanocytes, with resultant hyperpigmentation of the skin, particularly of sun-exposed areas and at pressure points, such as the neck, elbows, knees and knuckles. Decreased mineralocorticoid activity in patients with primary adrenal insufficiency results in potassium retention and sodium loss, with consequent hyperkalaemia, hyponatraemia, volume depletion and hypotension. Hypoglycaemia may occasionally occur as a result of glucocorticoid deficiency and impaired gluconeogenesis. Stresses such as infections, trauma or surgical procedures in such patients can precipitate an acute adrenal crisis, manifested by intractable vomiting, abdominal pain, hypotension, coma and vascular collapse. Death occurs rapidly unless corticosteroid therapy begins

pathology

immediately. More than 90% of all cases are attributable to one of four disorders: autoimmune adrenalitis, TB, the acquired immune deficiency syndrome (AIDS) or metastatic cancers.

3.89

Answer: E

Several epidemiological studies suggest that the use of aspirin and other NSAIDs exerts a protective effect against colon cancer. In the Nurses' Health Study, women who used four to six tablets of aspirin/day for 10 years or more had a decreased incidence of colon cancer. Two recent studies have revealed that aspirin reduces the risk of recurrent adenomas in patients with previous colorectal carcinomas or adenomas. The mechanism of such chemoprevention is not fully understood, but it is probably mediated by inhibition of cyclo-oxygenase-2 (COX-2). This enzyme is over-expressed in neoplastic epithelium and seems to regulate angiogenesis and apoptosis. On the basis of these findings, the US Food and Drug Administration (FDA) has approved the use of COX-2 inhibitors as chemopreventive agents in patients with the familial adenomatous polyposis syndrome.

3.90

Answer: D

Povidone–iodine is iodine complexed with povidone (polyvinyl-pyrrolidone). The compound is soluble in water, forming a golden-brown solution. Similar to iodine, the solution of the iodine complex is bactericidal and fungicidal. However, unlike solutions of iodine, it is non-staining. The antiseptic action of povidone–iodine solutions is the result of the available iodine present in the complex. It acts by oxidation/substitution of free iodine.

3.91

Answer: B

The term 'benign' refers to a tumour, condition or growth that is not cancerous. This means that it is localised and has not spread to other parts of the body or invaded and destroyed nearby tissue. In general, a benign tumour is usually not harmful and benign tumours usually grow slowly and are well encapsulated and well differentiated. They can usually be removed and in most cases they do not recur. However, if a benign tumour is big enough, the size and weight can press on nearby organs, blood vessels and nerves and thus cause problems.

Malignant neoplasms, in contrast, range from well differentiated to undifferentiated. Malignant neoplasms composed of undifferentiated cells are said to be anaplastic. Lack of differentiation, or anaplasia, is considered a hallmark of malignant transformation. Anaplasia literally means 'to form backward', implying a reversion from a high level of differentiation to a lower level. Lack of differentiation, or anaplasia, is marked by the following:

- Pleomorphism: both the cells and the nuclei characteristically display pleomorphism – variation in size and shape. Cells may be found that are many times larger than their neighbours, and other cells may be extremely small and appear primitive.
- Abnormal nuclear morphology: characteristically the nuclei contain an abundance of DNA and are extremely dark staining (hyperchromatic). The nuclei are disproportionately large for the cell, and the nucleus:cytoplasm ratio may approach 1:1 instead of the normal 1:4 or 1:6. The nuclear shape is very variable, and the chromatin is often coarsely clumped and distributed along the nuclear membrane. Large nucleoli are usually present in these nuclei.
- Mitoses: compared with benign tumours and some well-differentiated malignant neoplasms, undifferentiated tumours usually possess large numbers of mitoses, reflecting the higher proliferative activity of the parenchymal cells. The presence of mitoses does not, however, necessarily indicate that a tumour is malignant or that the tissue is neoplastic. Many normal tissues

pathology

exhibiting rapid turnover, such as bone marrow, have numerous mitoses, and non-neoplastic proliferations such as hyperplasias contain many cells in mitosis. More important as a morphological feature of malignant neoplasia are atypical, bizarre mitotic figures, sometimes producing tripolar, quadripolar or multipolar spindles.

- Loss of polarity: in addition to the cytological abnormalities, the orientation of anaplastic cells is markedly disturbed (ie they lose normal polarity). Sheets or large masses of tumour cells grow in an anarchic, disorganised fashion.

- Other changes: another feature of anaplasia is the formation of tumour giant cells, some possessing only a single huge polymorphic nucleus and others having two or more nuclei. These giant cells are not to be confused with inflammatory Langhans' or foreign body giant cells, which are derived from macrophages and contain many small, normal-appearing nuclei. In the cancer giant cell, the nuclei are hyperchromatic and large in relation to the cell.

Last but not least malignant tumours are locally invasive and frequently metastasise.

3.92

Answer: E

Rheumatic fever (RF) is an acute, immunologically mediated, multisystem inflammatory disease that occurs a few weeks after an episode of group A streptococcal pharyngitis. Acute rheumatic carditis during the active phase of RF may progress to chronic rheumatic heart disease. The most important consequence of RF is chronic valvular deformities, characterised principally by deforming fibrotic valvular disease (particularly mitral stenosis), which produces permanent dysfunction and severe, sometimes fatal, cardiac problems decades later. During acute RF, focal inflammatory lesions are found in various tissues. They are most distinctive within the heart, where they are called Aschoff's bodies. They consist of foci of swollen eosinophilic collagen surrounded by lymphocytes (primarily T cells), occasional plasma cells and plump macrophages called Anitschkow's cells (pathognomonic for RF). These distinctive cells have abundant cytoplasm and central round-to-ovoid nuclei in which the chromatin is disposed in a central, slender, wavy ribbon (hence the designation 'caterpillar cells'). Some of the larger macrophages become multinucleated to form Aschoff's giant cells. During acute RF, diffuse inflammation and Aschoff's bodies may be found in any of the three layers of the heart – pericardium, myocardium or endocardium – hence the lesion's name pancarditis. In the pericardium, the inflammation is accompanied by a fibrinous or serofibrinous pericardial exudate, described as a 'bread-and-butter' pericarditis, which generally resolves without sequelae. The myocardial involvement – myocarditis – takes the form of scattered Aschoff's bodies within the interstitial connective tissue, often perivascular.

Ferruginous bodies are iron-coated asbestos particles seen in pulmonary asbestosis. Foamy macrophages are lipid-laden macrophages seen in an atherosclerotic plaque and are not seen in rheumatic fever. Langhans' giant cells are seen in tuberculous granuloma. Pyogenic granuloma is a polypoid form of capillary haemangioma that occurs as a rapidly growing exophytic red nodule attached by a stalk to the skin and gingival or oral mucosa.

3.93

Answer: D

The induction and regulation of immune responses involve multiple interactions among lymphocytes, monocytes, inflammatory cells (eg neutrophils) and endothelial cells. Many such interactions depend on cell-to-cell contact; however, many interactions and effector functions are mediated by short-acting soluble mediators, called cytokines. This term includes the previously designated lymphokines (lymphocyte derived), monokines (monocyte derived) and several other polypeptides that regulate immunological, inflammatory and reparative host responses. Molecularly defined cytokines are called interleukins, implying that they mediate communications between

pathology

leukocytes. Most cytokines have a wide spectrum of effects and some are produced by several different cell types. The following list provides the major effects of various interleukins:

- IL-1: secreted by macrophages; induces acute-phase reaction
- IL-2: secreted by T cells, stimulates growth and differentiation of T-cell response; potential for immunotherapy to treat cancer
- IL-3: secreted by T cells, stimulates bone marrow stem cells
- IL-4: involved in proliferation of B cells, and the development of T cells and mast cells; important role in allergic responses
- IL-5: role in stimulation of B cells, eosinophil production and IgA production
- IL-6: secreted by macrophages; induces acute-phase reaction
- IL-7: involved in B-, T- and NK (natural killer) cell survival, development and homeostasis
- IL-8: neutrophil chemotaxis
- IL-9: stimulates mast cells
- IL-10: inhibits Th1 (T-helper type 1 cell) cytokine production
- IL-11: acute-phase protein production
- IL-12: NK cell stimulation; Th1 cell induction
- IL-13: stimulates growth and differentiation of B cells, inhibits Th1 cells and the production of macrophage inflammatory cytokines
- IL-17: induces production of inflammatory cytokines
- IL-18: induces production of interferon-γ.

3.94

Answer: C

A leukocytosis is an increase in the number of circulating leukocytes. A neutrophilic leukocytosis (neutrophilia) typically occurs in response to acute bacterial infections, especially those caused by pyogenic organisms, eg streptococcal pneumonia. It is also seen in sterile inflammation caused by, for example, tissue necrosis (myocardial infarction, burns). All of the other conditions listed are associated with eosinophilia. The most common causes of eosinophilia are allergic diseases and parasitic infections. The parasitic infections that are associated with eosinophilia involve invasion of the tissues. In addition, there are several other causes of eosinophilia. The mnemonic for eosinophilia is 'worms, wheezes and weird diseases'. Hay fever and asthma are both caused by a type I immune injury (IgE mediated), in which eosinophilia occurs. *Ascaris* species cause a parasitic tissue infection (non-respiratory). 'Weird diseases' refers to a wide array of other conditions, including Hodgkin's disease, eosinophilic gastroenteritis, Loeffler's syndrome, pemphigus and dermatitis herpetiformis.

3.95

Answer: A

- *Streptococcus pneumoniae* is a Gram-positive organism that is flame shaped and seen characteristically as diplococci (ie in pairs) and capsulated. The organism grows on blood agar to form dome-shaped, centrally umbilicated colonies and produces a haemolysis of the RBCs.
- *Staphylococcus aureus* is not the correct answer because it is typically seen in clusters under the microscope when Gram stained and also its colonies are raised and not dome shaped. It produces β haemolysis on blood agar rather than a haemolysis.
- *Klebsiella pneumoniae* is also unlikely because it is a Gram-negative rather than a Gram-positive organism. It will be seen under the microscope as rods rather then cocci.
- *Corynebacterium diphtheriae* causes only an upper respiratory tract infection. It does not cause pneumonia so it cannot be brought up in the sputum.
- *Mycoplasma pneumoniae* can cause pneumonia but is incorrect because it does not take up Gram stain and also does not grow on blood agar.

pathology

3.96

Answer: E

Infiltrating ductal adenocarcinoma of the pancreas, more commonly known as 'pancreatic cancer,' is primarily a disease in elderly people, 80% of cases occurring between the ages of 60 and 80. It is more common in black than in white individuals, and it is slightly more common in individuals of Jewish decent. The strongest environmental influence is smoking, which is believed to double the risk of pancreatic cancer. Other associated aetiological factors include alcohol, chronic pancreatitis, consumption of a diet rich in fats and diabetes mellitus. About 60% of cancers of the pancreas arise in the head of the gland, 15% in the body and 5% in the tail; in 20%, the neoplasm diffusely involves the entire gland. The *K-RAS* gene (chromosome 12p) is the most frequently altered oncogene in pancreatic cancer. This oncogene is activated by point mutation in 80–90% of pancreatic cancers.

Carcinomas of the pancreas remain silent until their extension impinges on some other structure. Pain is usually the first symptom, but by the time pain appears these cancers are usually beyond cure. Obstructive jaundice is associated with most cases of carcinoma of the head of the pancreas, but it rarely draws attention to the invasive cancer soon enough. Weight loss, anorexia, and generalised malaise and weakness tend to be signs of advanced disease. Migratory thrombophlebitis, known as Trousseau's sign, occurs in about 10% of patients and is attributable to the elaboration of platelet-aggregating factors and pro-coagulants from the tumour or its necrotic products. Despite the tendency of lesions of the head of the pancreas to obstruct the biliary system, less than 20% of pancreatic cancers overall are resectable at the time of diagnosis. The 5-year survival rate is dismal, < 5%.

3.97

Answer: E

More than one system is used for staging colorectal cancer. These include Dukes', Astler–Coller and AJCC/TNM systems. The AJCC system (also called the TNM system) describes stages using Roman numerals I–IV. Both Dukes' system and the Astler–Coller system use A–C; the Astler–Coller system adds stage D and has more subdivisions.

The AJCC/TNM system describes the extent of the primary tumour (T), the absence or presence of metastasis to nearby lymph nodes (N), and the absence or presence of distant metastasis (M).

T categories for colorectal cancer

T categories of colorectal cancer describe the extent of spread through the layers that form the wall of the colon and rectum. These layers, from the inner to the outer, include the lining (*mucosa*), the fibrous tissue beneath this muscle layer (*submucosa*), a thick layer of muscle that contracts to force the contents of the intestines along (*muscularis propria*) and the thin outermost layers of connective tissue (*subserosa and serosa*) that cover most of the colon but not the rectum.

T_x: no description of the tumour's extent is possible because of incomplete information.

T_{is}: the cancer is in the earliest stage. It has not grown beyond the mucosa (inner layer) of the colon or rectum. This stage is also known as carcinoma in situ or intramucosal carcinoma.

T_1: the cancer has grown through the mucosa and extends into the submucosa.

T_2: the cancer has grown through the submucosa and extends into the muscularis propria.

T_3: the cancer has grown completely through the muscularis propria into the subserosa, but not to any neighbouring organs or tissues.

T_4: the cancer has spread completely through the wall of the colon or rectum into nearby tissues or organs.

N categories for colorectal cancer

N categories indicate whether or not the cancer has spread to nearby lymph nodes and, if so, how many lymph nodes are involved.

N_x: no description of lymph node involvement is possible because of incomplete information.

N_0: no lymph node involvement is found.

N_1: cancer cells found in one to three nearby lymph nodes.

N_2: cancer cells found in four or more nearby lymph nodes.

M categories for colorectal cancer

M categories indicate whether or not the cancer has spread to distant organs, such as the liver, lungs or distant lymph nodes.

M_x: no description of distant spread is possible because of incomplete information.

M_0: no distant spread is seen.

M_1: distant spread is present.

Stage grouping

Once a patient's T, N and M categories have been determined, usually after surgery, this information is combined in a process called *stage grouping* to determine the stage, expressed in Roman numerals from stage I (the least advanced stage) to stage IV (the most advanced stage). The following guide illustrates how TNM categories are grouped together into stages:

Stage 0 (T_{IS} N_0 M_0): the cancer is in the earliest stage. It has not grown beyond the inner layer (mucosa) of the colon or rectum. This stage is also known as carcinoma in situ or intramucosal carcinoma.

Stage I (T_1 N_0 M_0, or T2 N_0 M_0): the cancer has grown through the mucosa into the submucosa *or* it may also have grown into the muscularis propria, but it has not spread into nearby lymph nodes or distant sites.

Stage IIA (T_3 N_0 M_0): the cancer has grown through the wall of the colon or rectum into the outermost layers. It has not yet spread to the nearby lymph nodes or distant sites.

Stage IIB (T_4 N_0 M_0): the cancer has grown through the wall of the colon or rectum into other nearby tissues or organs. It has not yet spread to the nearby lymph nodes or distant sites.

Stage IIIA (T_{1-2} N_1 M_0): the cancer has grown through the mucosa into the submucosa *or* it may also have grown into the muscularis propria, and it has spread to one to three nearby lymph nodes but not distant sites.

Stage IIIB (T_{3-4} N_1 M_0): the cancer has grown through the wall of the colon or rectum *or* into other nearby tissues or organs and has spread

pathology

to one to three nearby lymph nodes but not distant sites.

Stage IIIC (any T N_2 M_0): the cancer can be any T but has spread to four or more nearby lymph nodes but not distant sites.

Stage IV (any T any N M_1): the cancer can be any T, any N, but has spread to distant sites such as the liver, lung, peritoneum (the membrane lining the abdominal cavity) or ovary.

As the patient in this scenario has got more than four nodes (N_2) but no distant metastases he has stage IIIC disease.

3.98

Answer: B

Cancer antigen (CA)-27.29 is a monoclonal antibody to a glycoprotein (MUC1) that is present on the apical surface of normal epithelial cells. CA-27.29 is highly associated with breast cancer, although levels are elevated in several other malignancies including colon, gastric, hepatic, lung, pancreatic, ovarian and prostate cancers. It also can be found in patients with benign disorders of the breast, liver and kidney, and in patients with ovarian cysts. However, CA-27.29 levels higher than 100 U/ml are rare in benign conditions. As a result of superior sensitivity and specificity, CA-27.29 has supplanted CA-15-3 as the preferred tumour marker in breast cancer. The CA-27.29 level is elevated in about a third of women with early stage breast cancer (stage I or II) and in two-thirds of women with late-stage disease (stage III or IV). CA-27.29 lacks predictive value in the earliest stages of breast cancer and thus has no role in screening for or diagnosing the malignancy. However, it is used most frequently to follow the response to therapy in patients with metastatic breast cancer. One trial in patients at high risk for recurrence of breast cancer (stage II or III) found that CA-27.29 was highly specific and sensitive in detecting preclinical metastasis. The average time from initial elevation of CA-27.29 to onset of symptoms was 5 months. As CA-27.29 testing may lead to prompt imaging of probable sites of metastasis, it may be possible to decrease morbidity through earlier institution of therapy.

Carcinoembryonic antigen (CEA), an oncofetal glycoprotein, is expressed in normal mucosal cells and over-expressed in

pathology

adenocarcinoma, especially colorectal cancer. CEA elevations also occur with other malignancies. Non-neoplastic conditions associated with elevated CEA levels include cigarette smoking, peptic ulcer disease, inflammatory bowel disease, pancreatitis, hypothyroidism, biliary obstruction and cirrhosis. Levels > 10 ng/ml are rarely caused by benign disease.

Elevated levels of CA-19-9, an intracellular adhesion molecule, occur primarily in patients with pancreatic and biliary tract cancers but have also been reported in patients with other malignancies. This tumour marker has a sensitivity and specificity of 80–90% for pancreatic cancer and a sensitivity of 60–70% for biliary tract cancer. Benign conditions such as cirrhosis, cholestasis, cholangitis and pancreatitis also result in CA-19-9 elevations, although values are usually < 1000 U/ml.

CA-125 is a glycoprotein normally expressed in coelomic epithelium during fetal development. This epithelium lines body cavities and envelopes the ovaries. Elevated CA-125 values are most often associated with epithelial ovarian cancer, although levels can also be increased in other malignancies. CA-125 levels are elevated in about 85% of women with ovarian cancer, but only 50% of those with stage I disease. Higher levels are associated with increasing bulk of disease and are highest in tumours with non-mucinous histology. AFP is the major protein of fetal serum but falls to an undetectable level after birth. The primary malignancies associated with AFP elevations are hepatocellular carcinoma and non-seminomatous germ cell tumours. Other gastrointestinal cancers occasionally cause elevations of AFP, but rarely to > 1000 ng/ml.

3.99

Answer: A

The catabolic phase immediately follows an insult and may last from 3 to 8 days after uncomplicated elective surgery. After severe stress, such as multiple trauma or thermal injury, this phase may persist for weeks. The catabolic phase is governed by the classic sympathoadrenal response. In the immediate period after an insult, metabolic demands increase and there is a mobilisation of protein to serve as a substrate for gluconeogenesis. Resting energy expenditure may increase dramatically depending on the severity of the insult. Urinary nitrogen excretion increases to levels greater than those seen in simple starvation and may exceed 20 g/day. Lipolysis and fatty acid oxidation are also increased. The normal response to insulin is lost and the patient becomes insulin resistant. The normal response of skeletal muscle to insulin is decreased by up to 50%.

3.100

Answer: D

Synovial fluid analysis is commonly performed to determine the cause of acute arthritis. It is of critical importance in establishing the diagnosis of septic arthritis and can be important in establishing a diagnosis of crystal-induced arthritis such as gout or pseudogout. The table below presents synovial fluid analysis findings in some common disorders causing arthritis.

Examination of synovial fluid

Suspected condition	Appearance	Viscosity	Cells (WBC/mm³)	Crystals	Biochemistry	Bacteriology
Normal	Clear yellow	High	< 200	–	As for plasma	–
Septic arthritis	Purulent	Low	> 100,000[a]	–	Glucose low	+
Tuberculous arthritis	Turbid	Low	2000–75,000	–	Glucose low	+
Rheumatoid arthritis	Cloudy	Low	2000–75,000	–	–	–
Gout[b]	Cloudy	Normal	2000–75,000	Urate	–	–
Pseudogout[c]	Cloudy	Normal	2000–75,000	CPPD	+	–
Osteoarthritis	Clear yellow	High	200–2000	–	–	–

[a]> 75% are polymorphonuclear leukocytes.

[b]The urate crystals in gout are thin, needle-shaped and negatively birefringent.

[c]The CPPD (calcium pyrophosphate dihydrate) crystals in pseudogout are rhomboid, often short and variable in shape, with weakly positive birefringence.

pathology

INDEX

(The number in bold indicates section and the number in italics indicates question number)